Mommy To Be: Activity Book for Pregnant Women

© 2023

By Dominique M. Williams

ISBN: 979-8-9874143-6-1

This Activity Book for Pregnant Women Belongs To:

_____

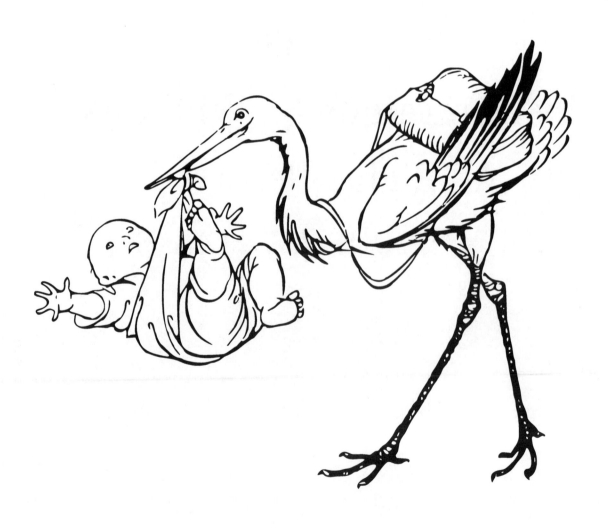

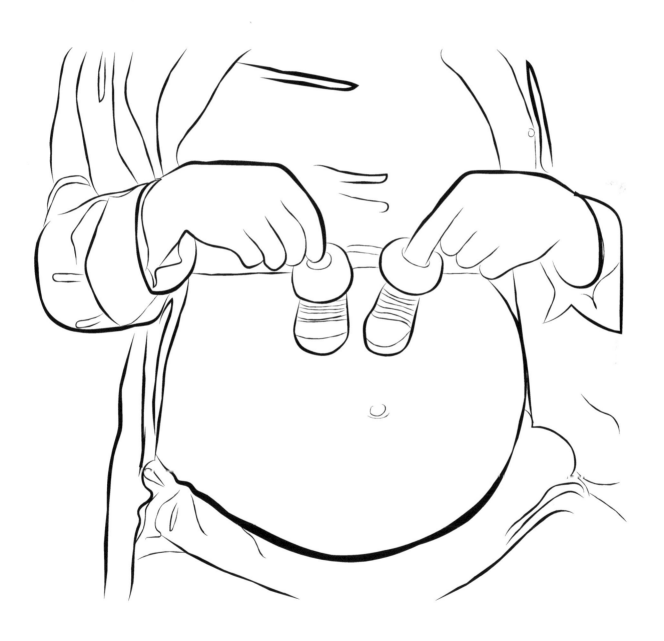

set

intentions

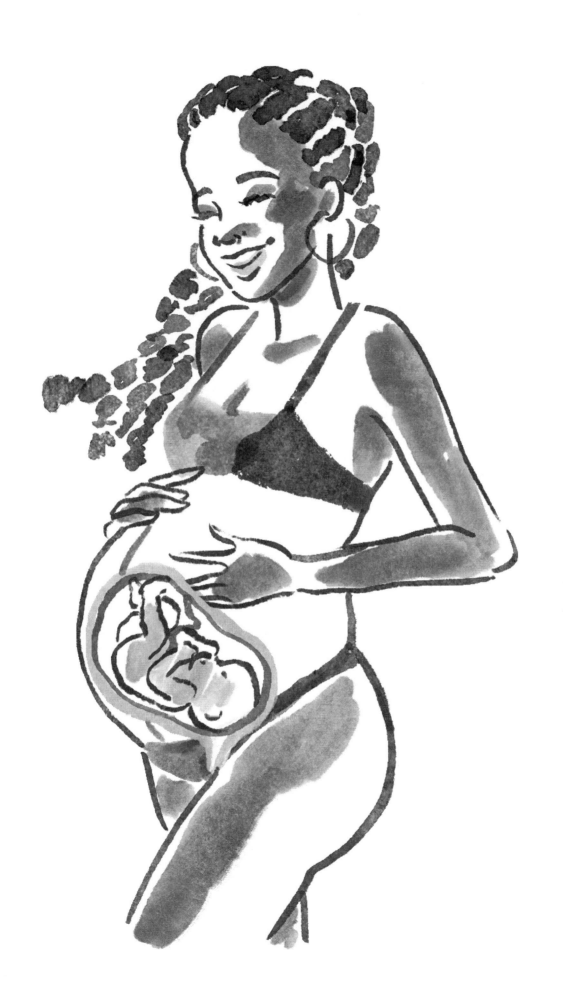

~ you're ~
amazing

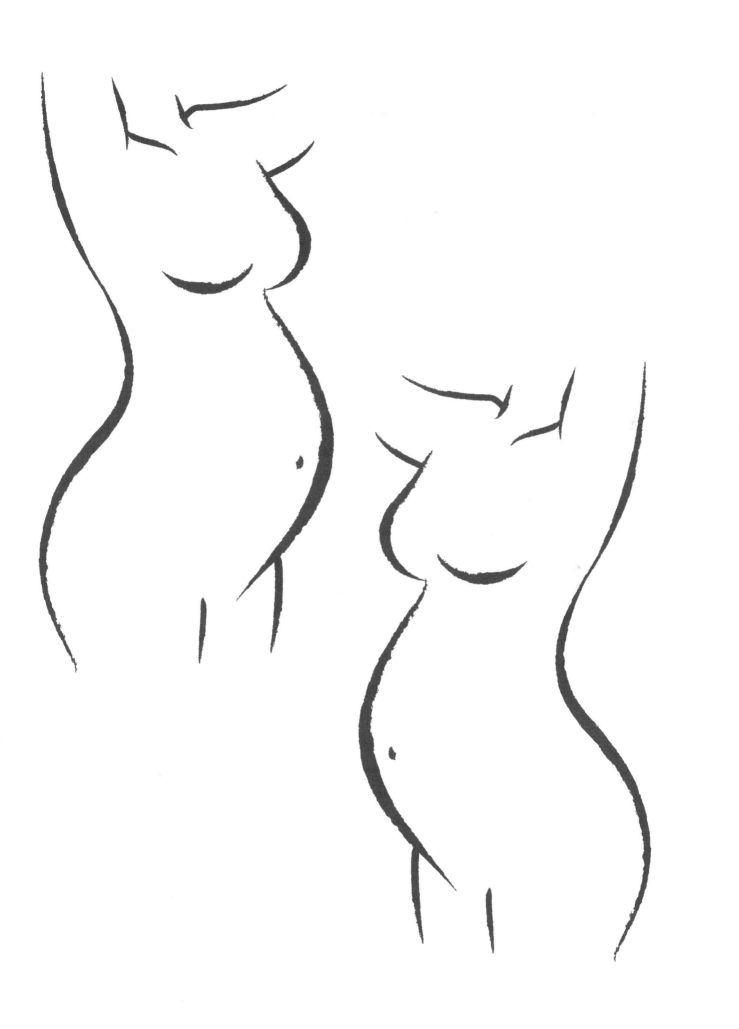

Who has been supportive during this pregnancy?

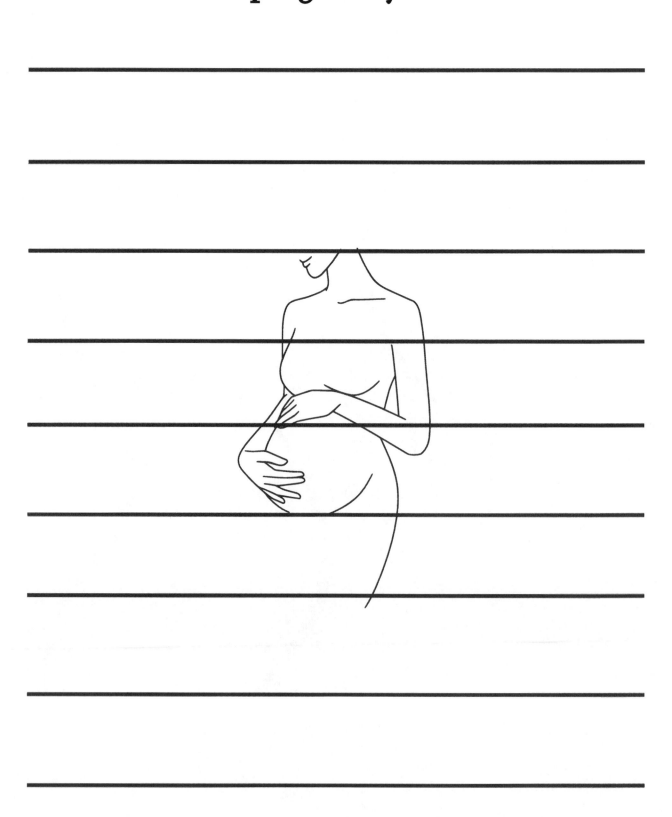

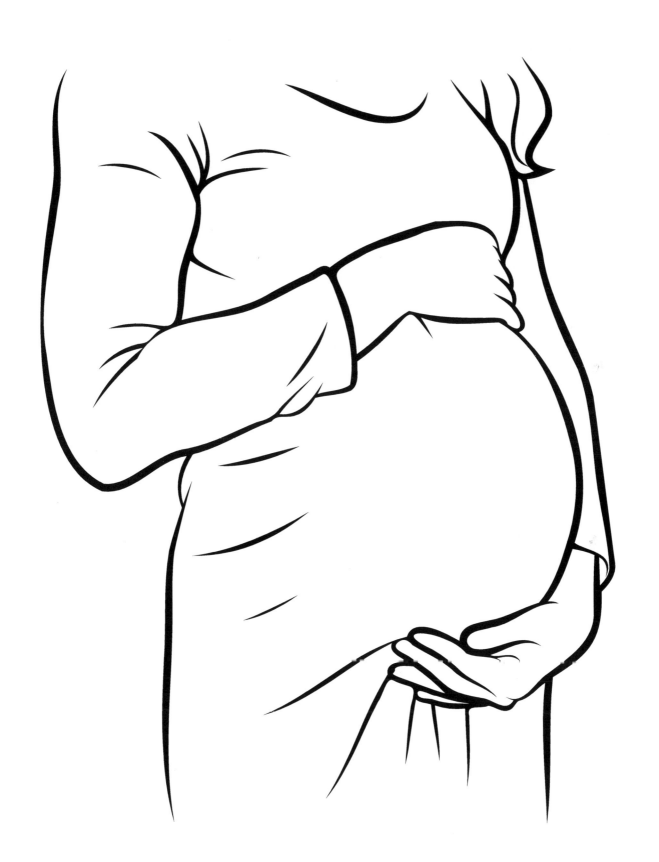

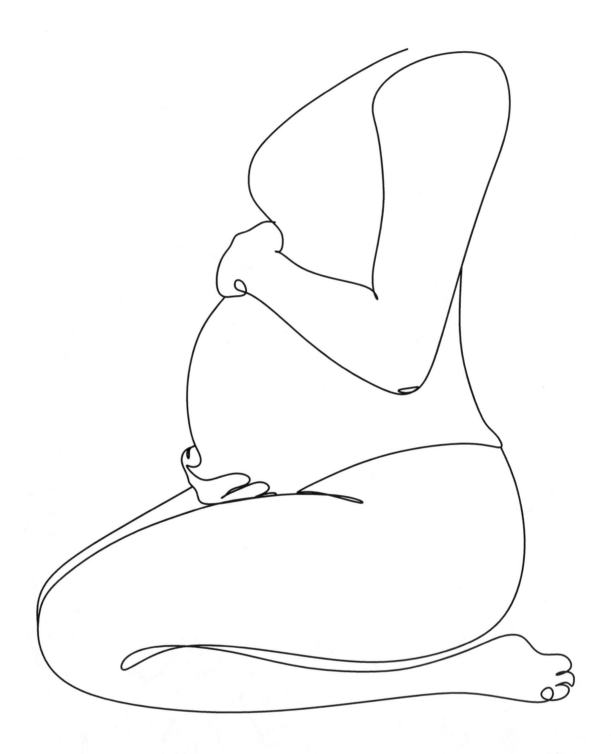

"As you cradle life within, remember to cradle yourself too."

Dominique M. Williams

In what ways would you like to be supported during this pregnancy?

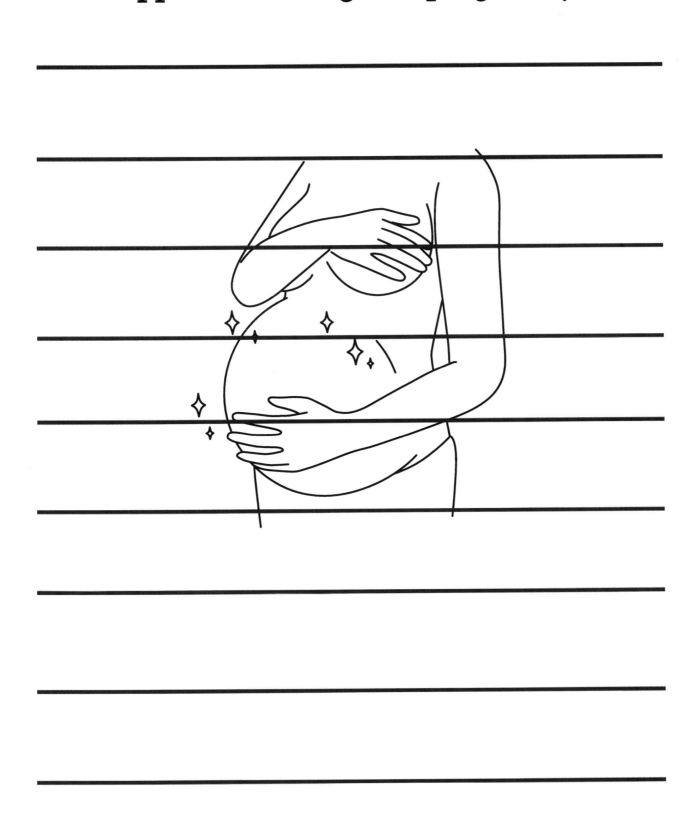

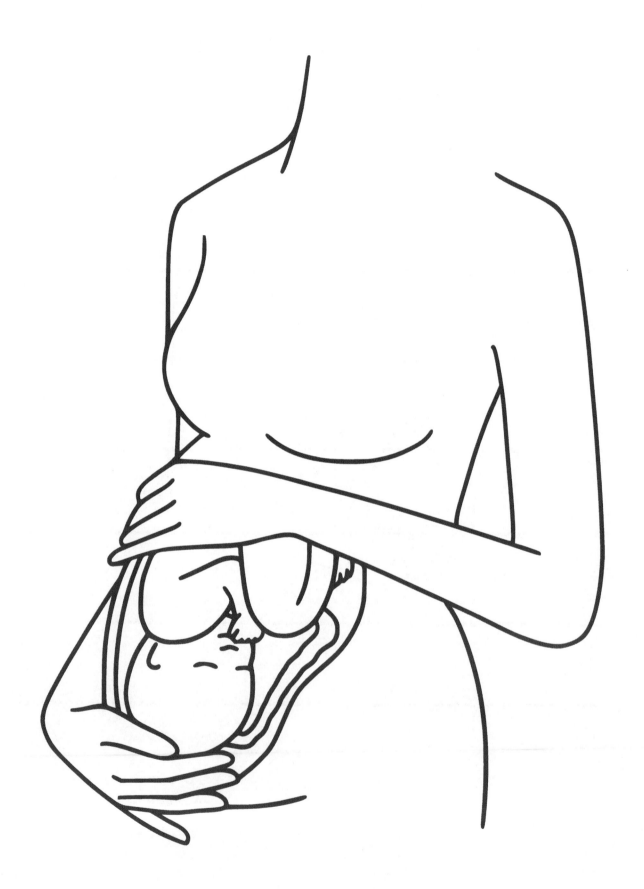

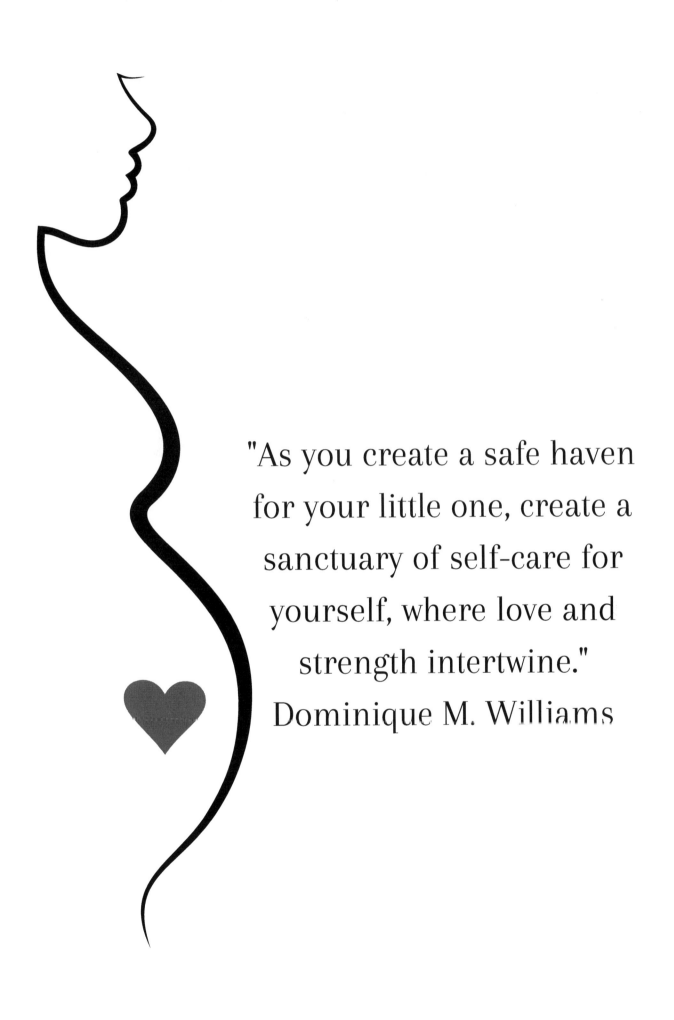

"As you create a safe haven for your little one, create a sanctuary of self-care for yourself, where love and strength intertwine."
Dominique M. Williams

How much have you been able to prioritize yourself and your needs during this pregnancy?

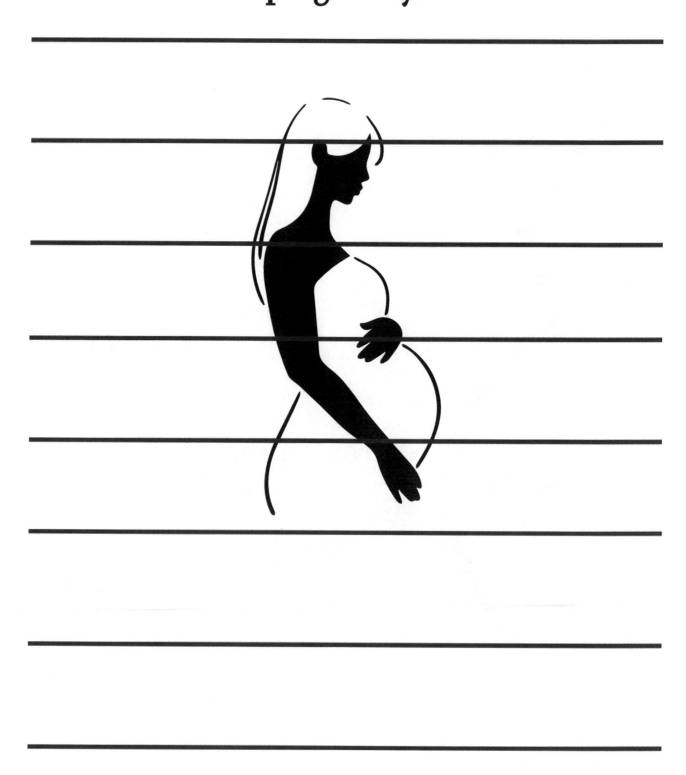

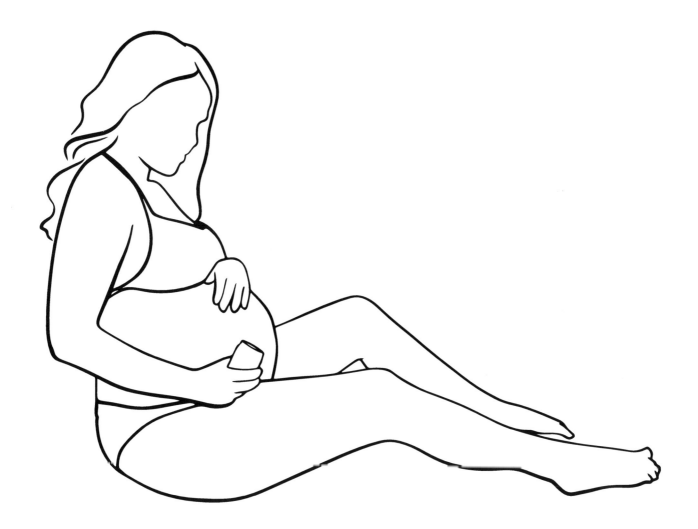

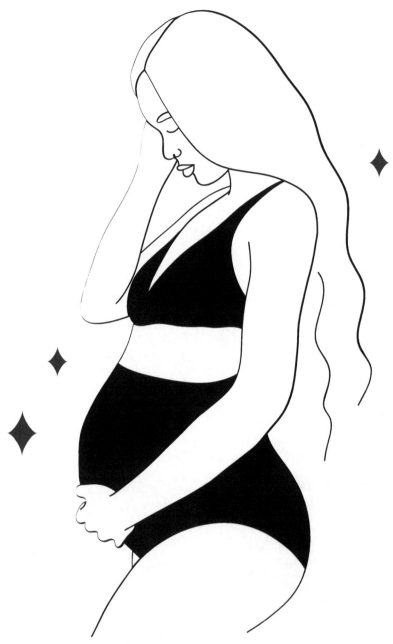

"Your body is a vessel of life, and your heart is its compass. Allow self-care to steer you towards the shores of tranquility."
Dominique M. Williams

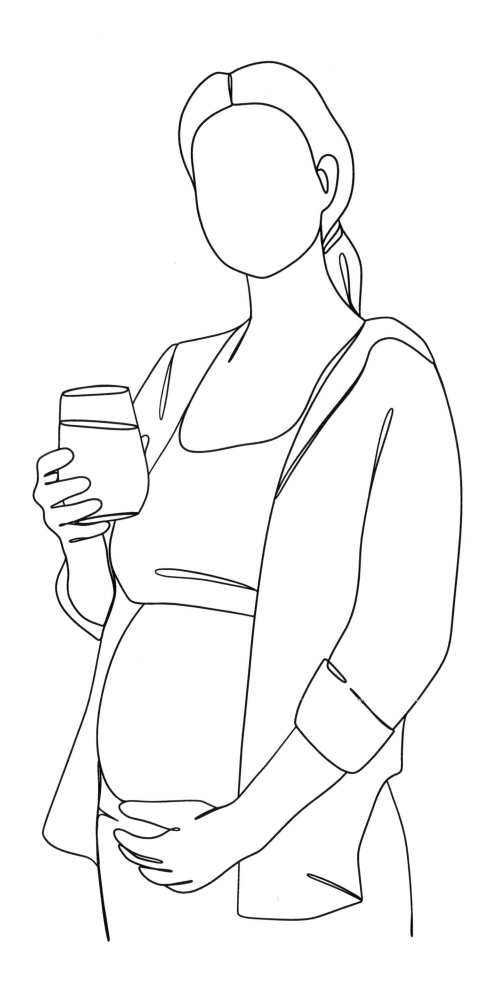

THiS
WiLL
PASS

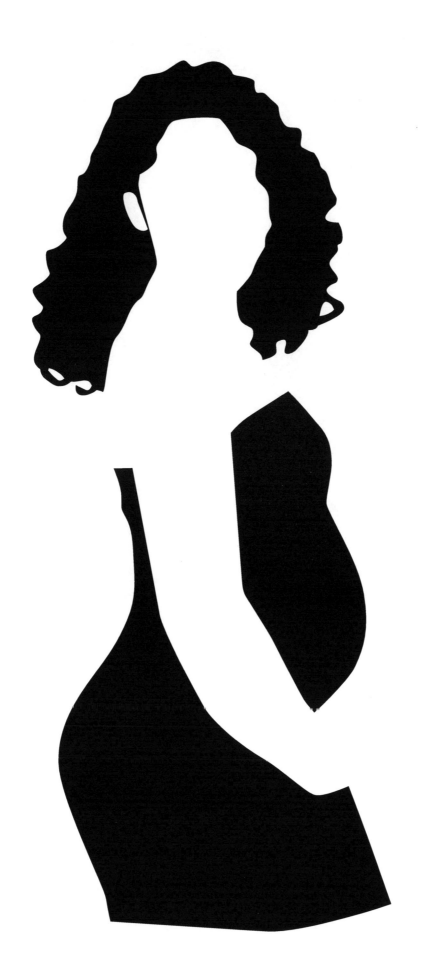

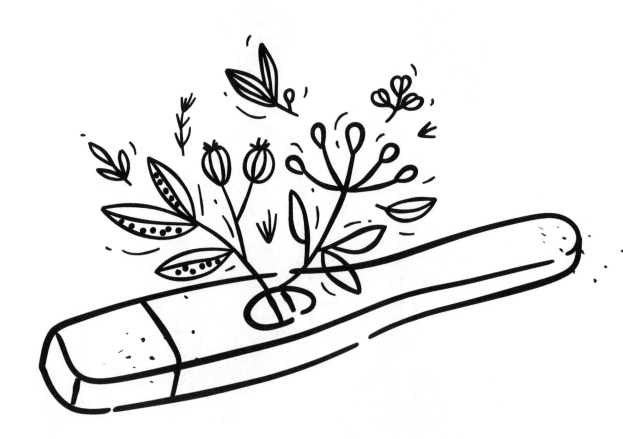

Your baby has began blooming.

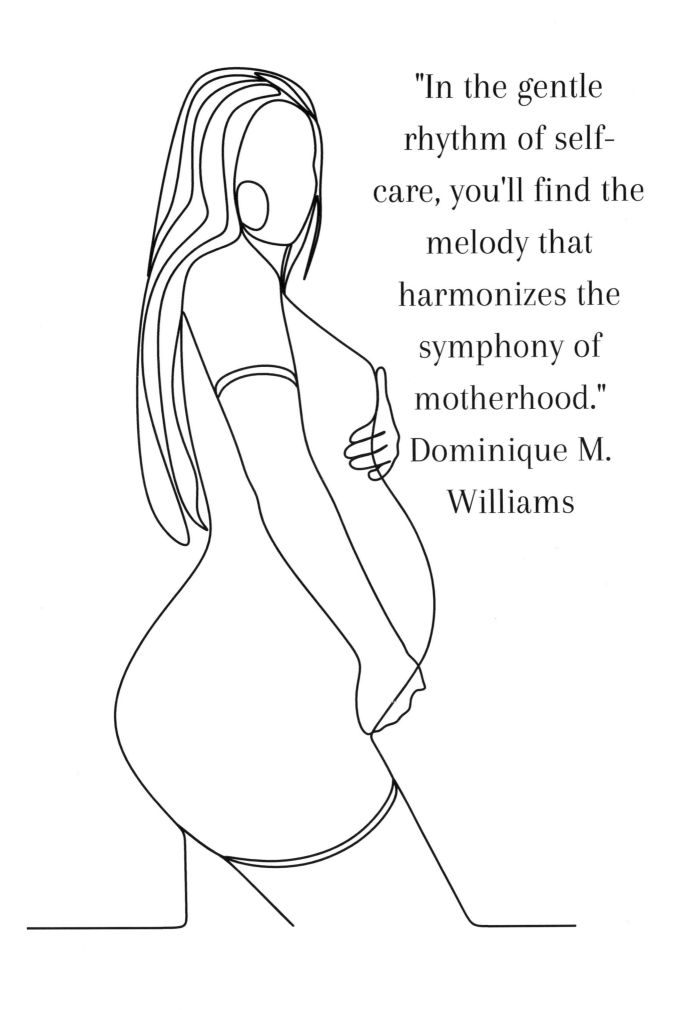

"In the gentle rhythm of self-care, you'll find the melody that harmonizes the symphony of motherhood."
Dominique M. Williams

Have you verbalized your needs & desires in your
relationships? (career, family, friends, significant other)

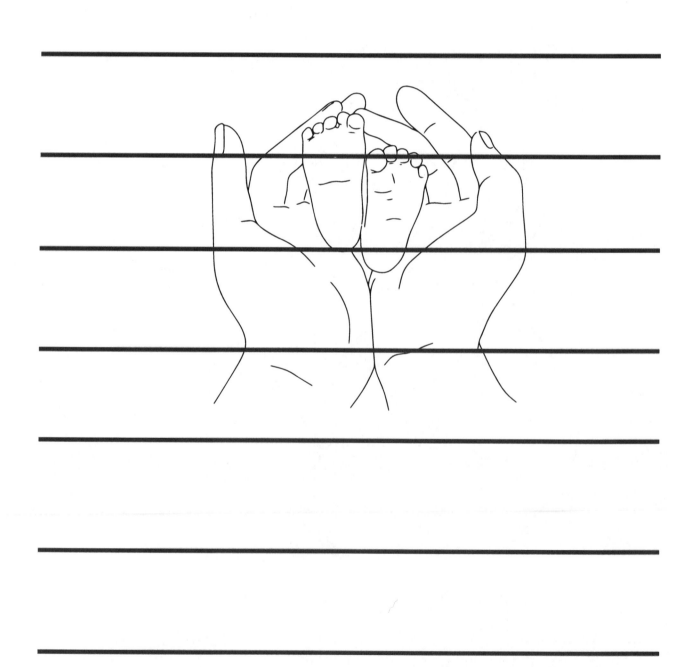

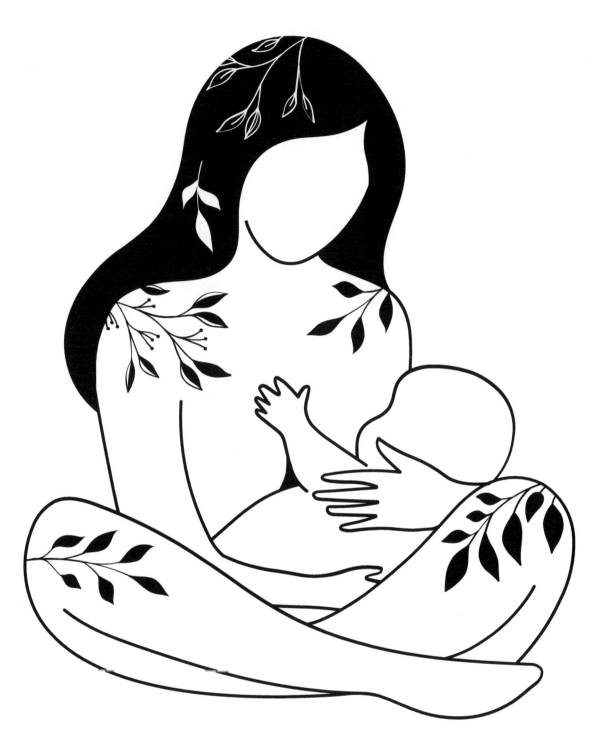

"Self-care is the key to keeping you and your baby's heart thriving and strong."
Dominique M. Williams

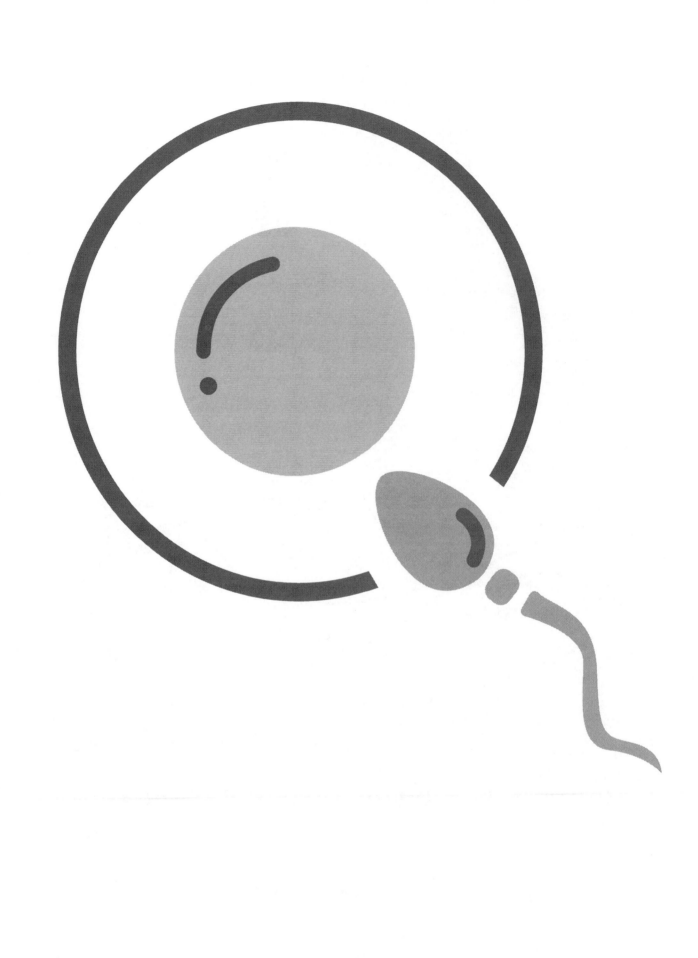

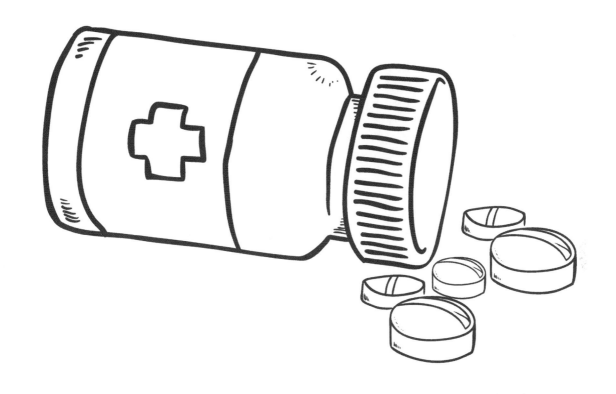

" Taking your prenatal vitamins, prescribed medications, and keeping your doctor appointments are extremely important for mom and baby.
Dominique M. Williams

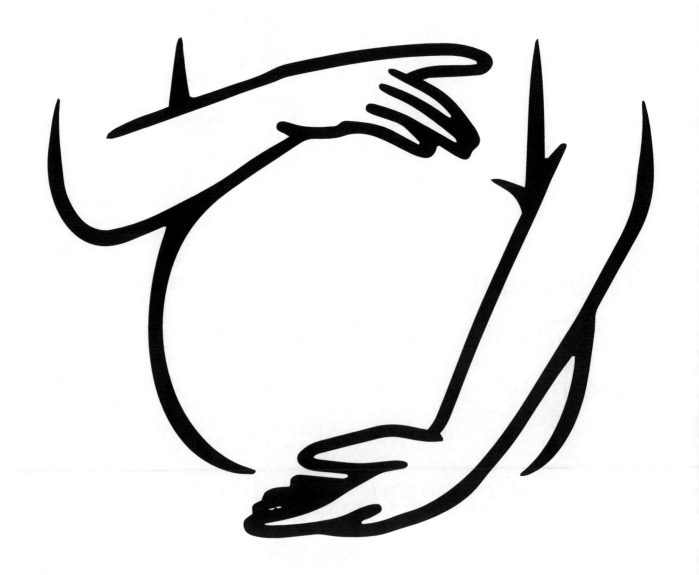

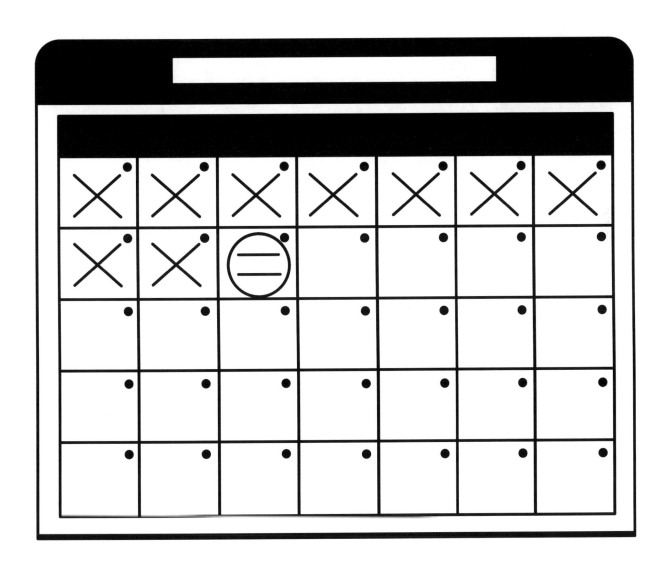

Were you tracking your ovulation days?

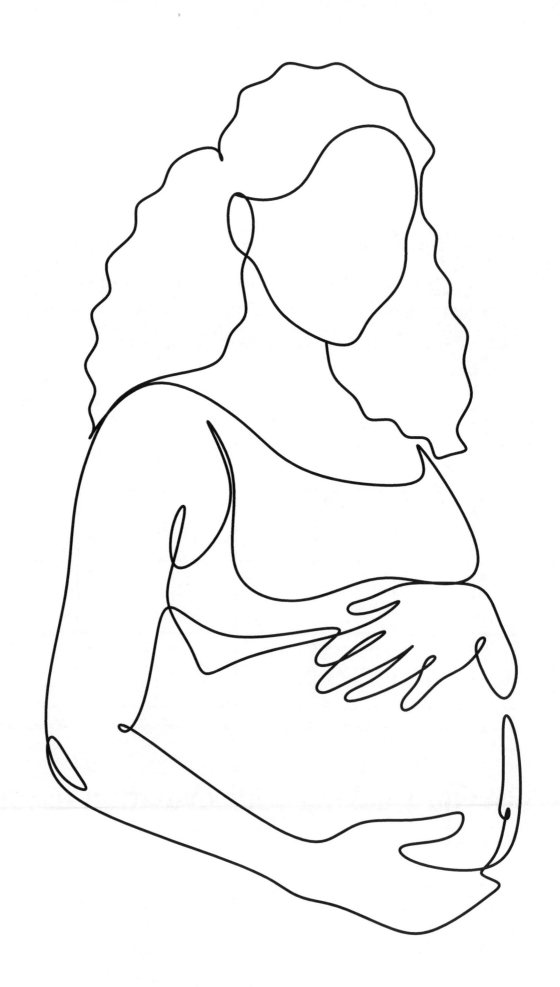

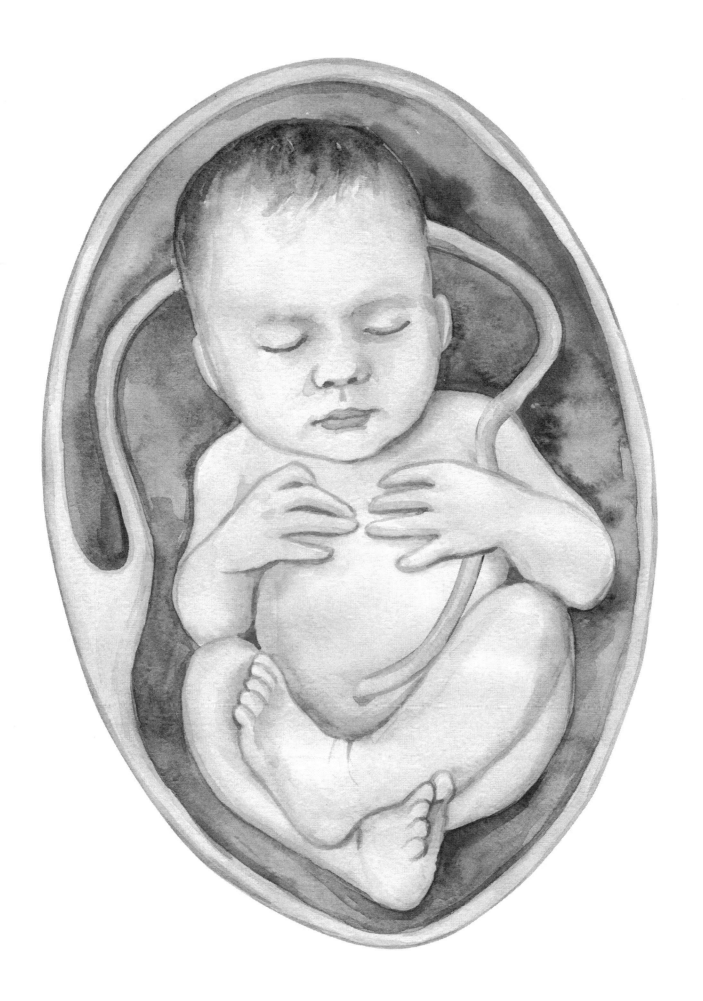

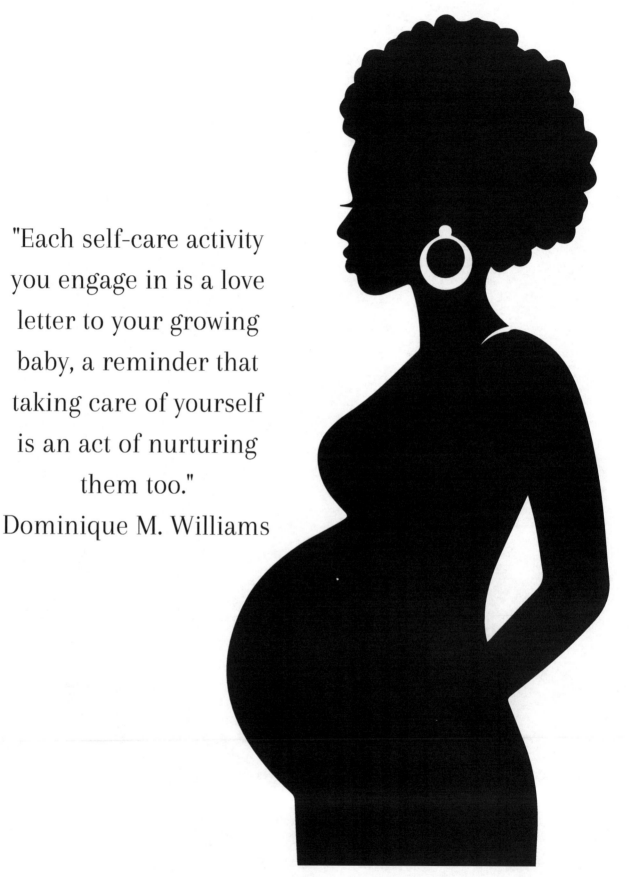

"Each self-care activity you engage in is a love letter to your growing baby, a reminder that taking care of yourself is an act of nurturing them too."
Dominique M. Williams

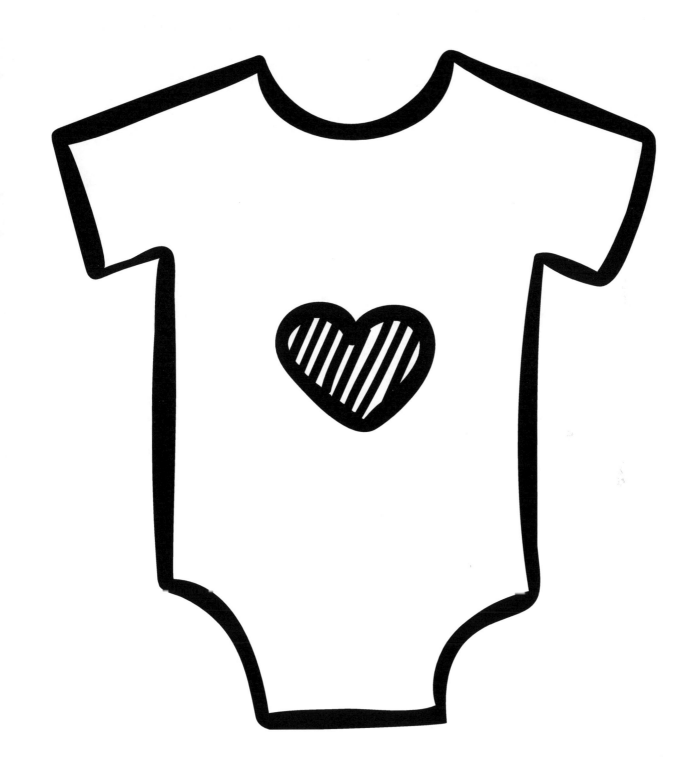

Once your bundle of joy arrives life as you currently know it will change. Where can you begin shifting to reclaim some time and energy for yourself.

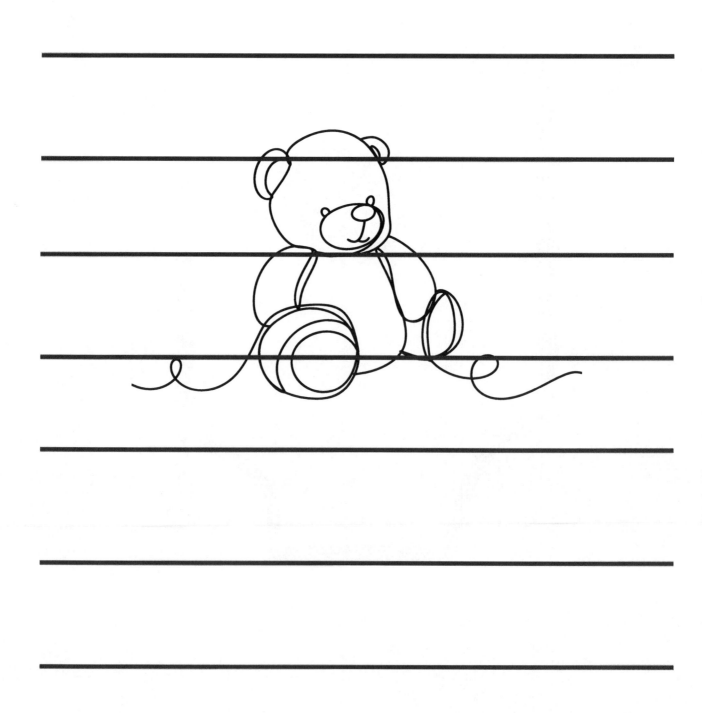

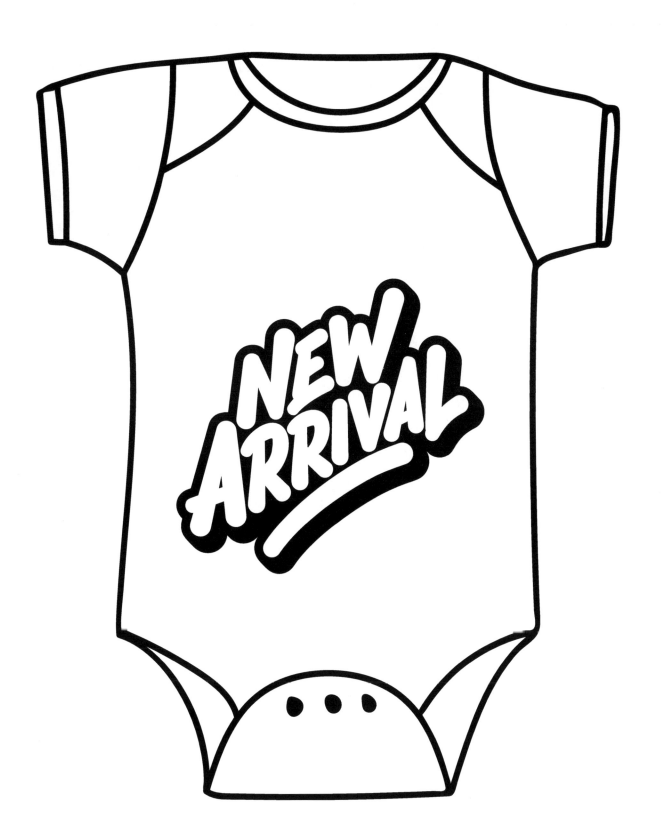

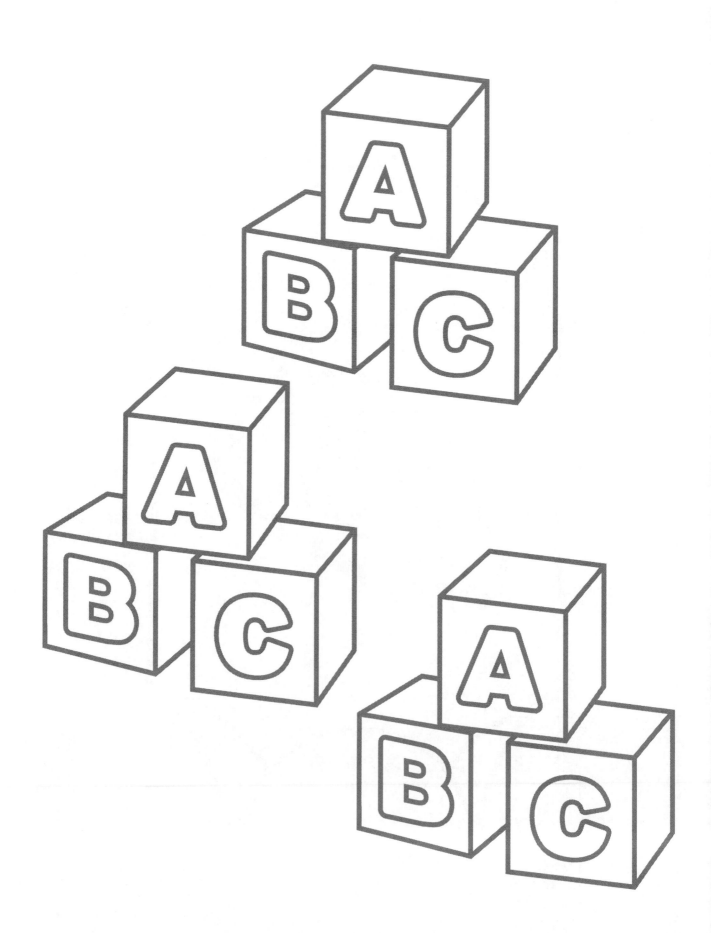

Have you decided if you'll breast feed or bottle feed your baby?

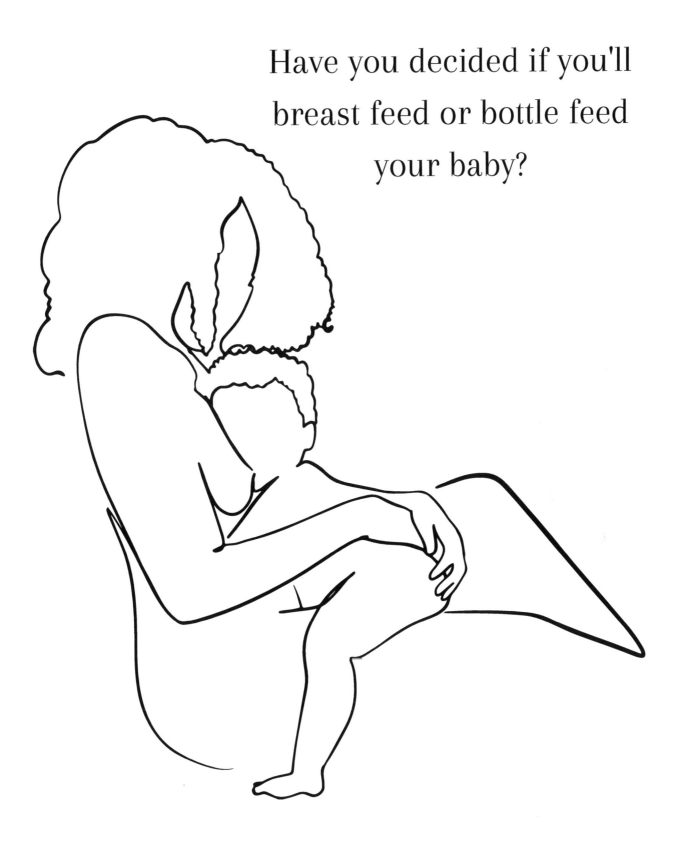

YOU ARE SO BEAUTIFUL

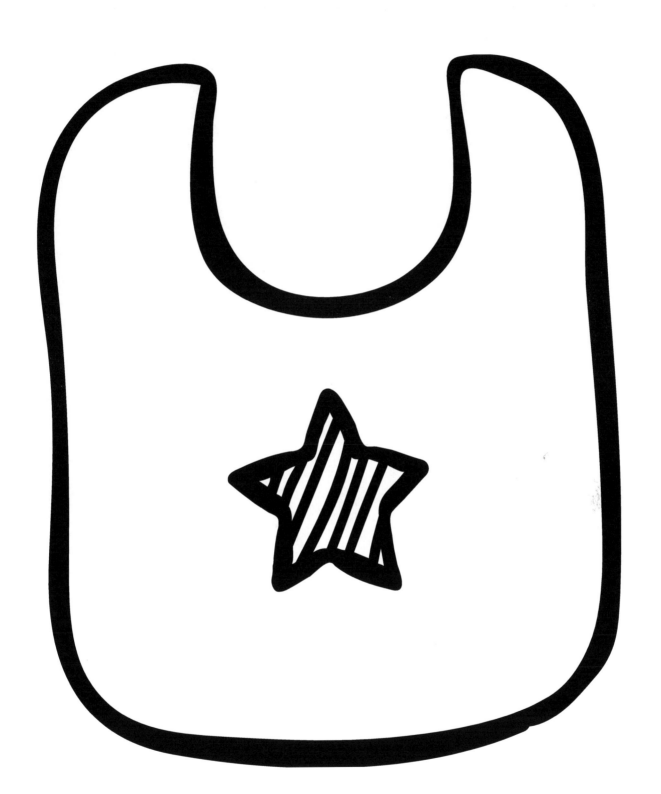

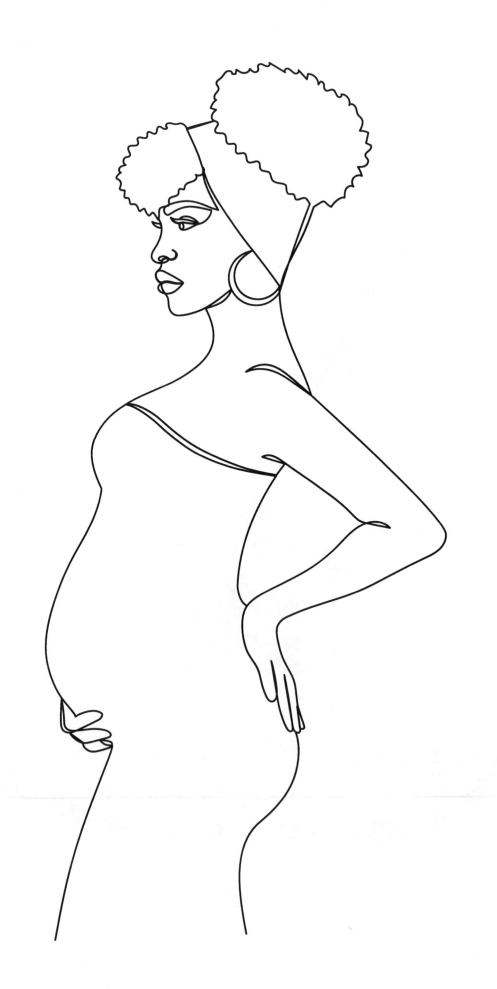

"Amongst the cravings and changes, remember to feed your soul."
Dominique M. Williams

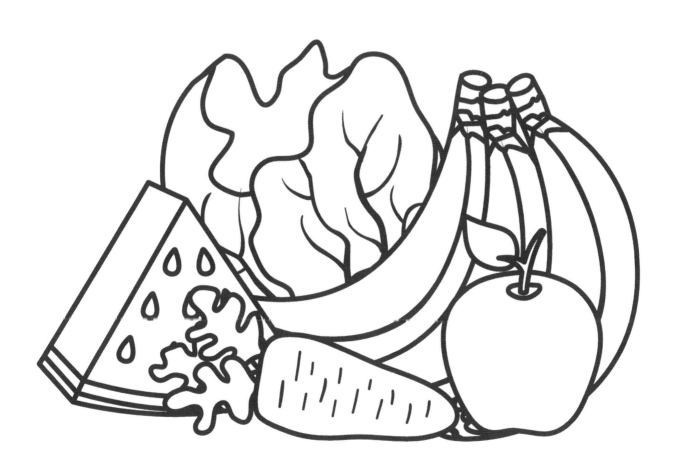

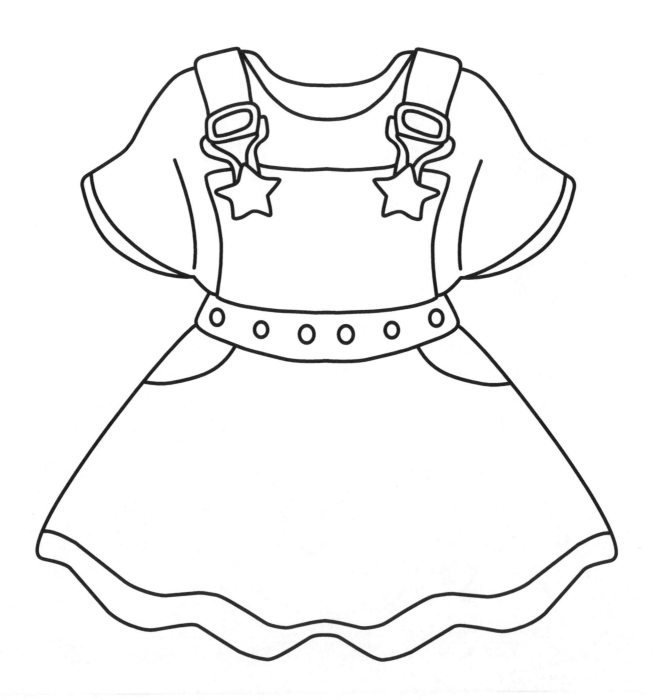

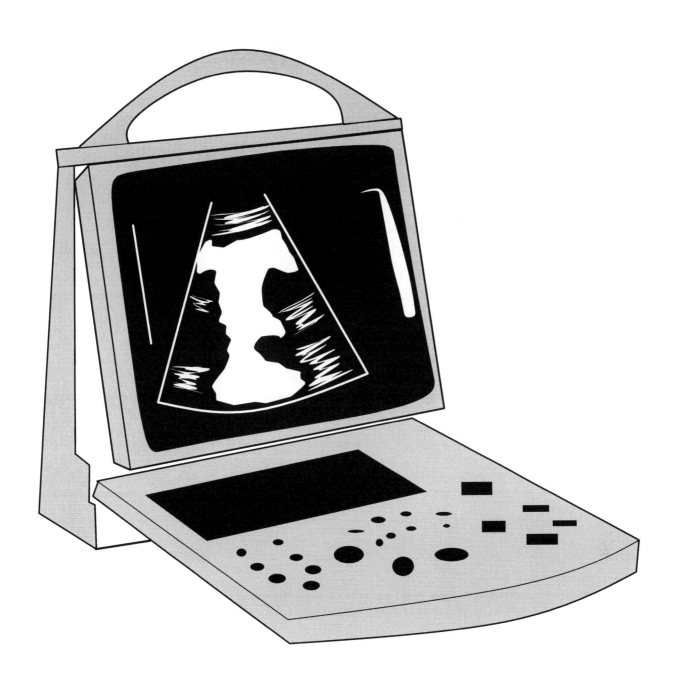

Ultrasound appointments are the best,
especially when you get to hear your little
one's heartbeat!

During this pregnancy have you spent time doing things that bring you joy? Make it a priority to implement something you love into your daily life.

_____

_____

_____

_____

_____

_____

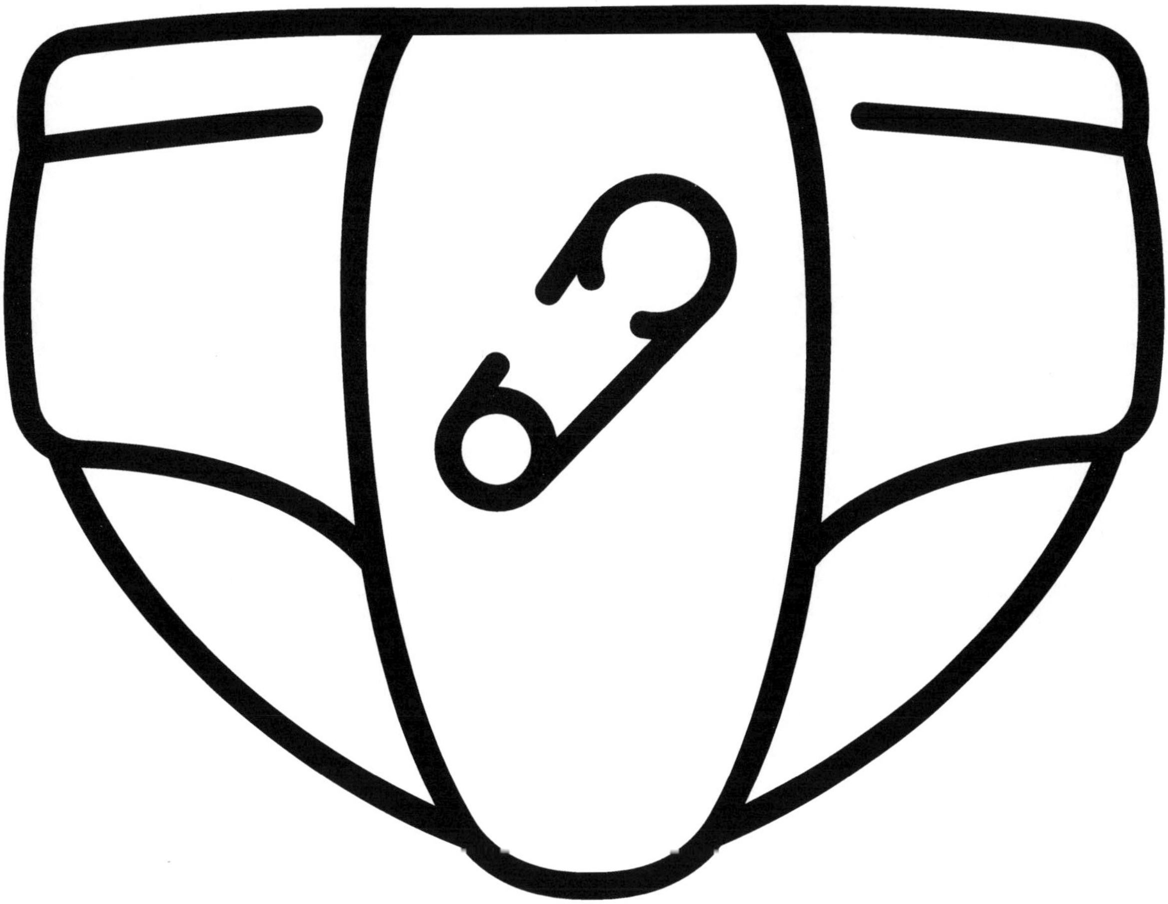

mommy to-be

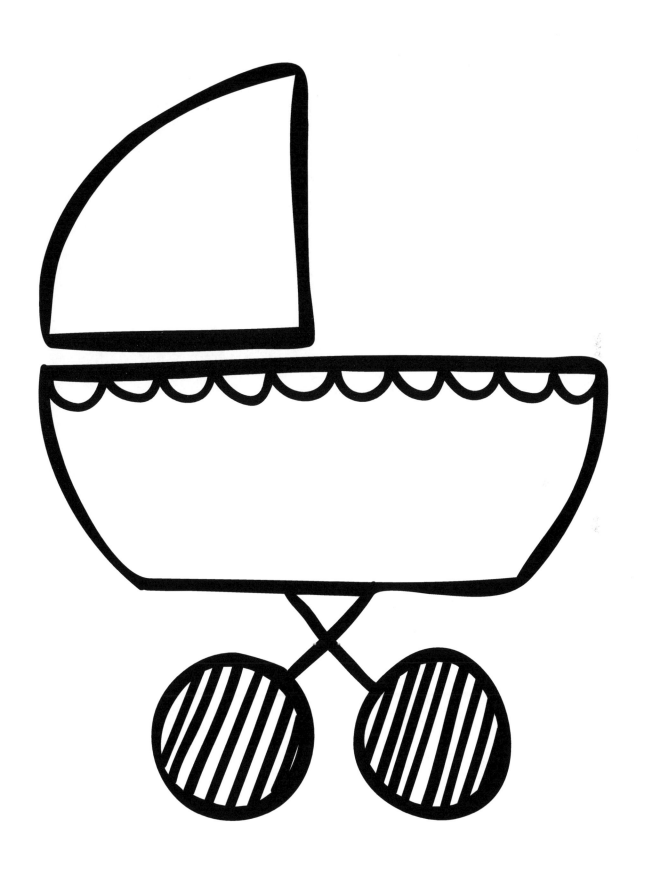

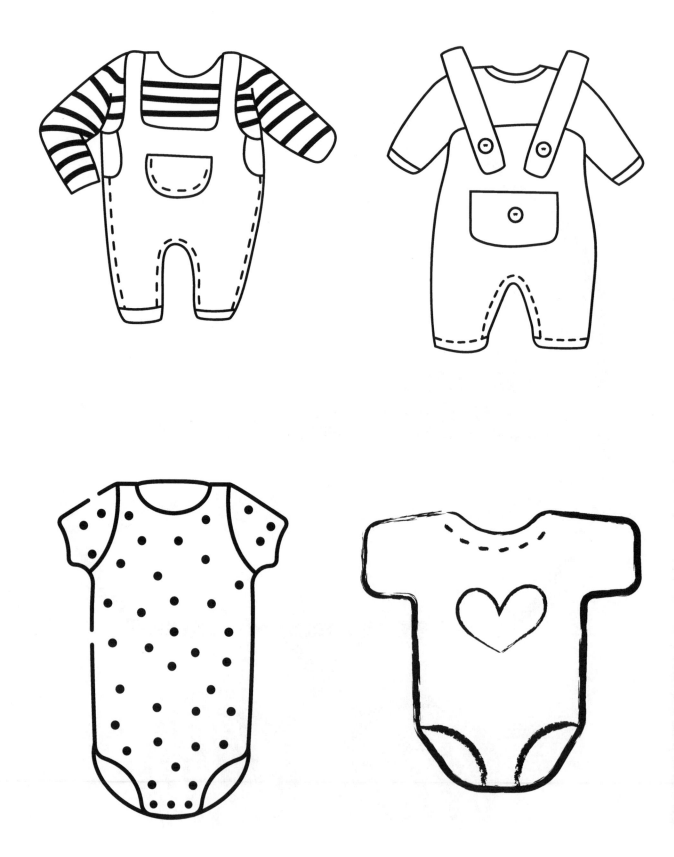

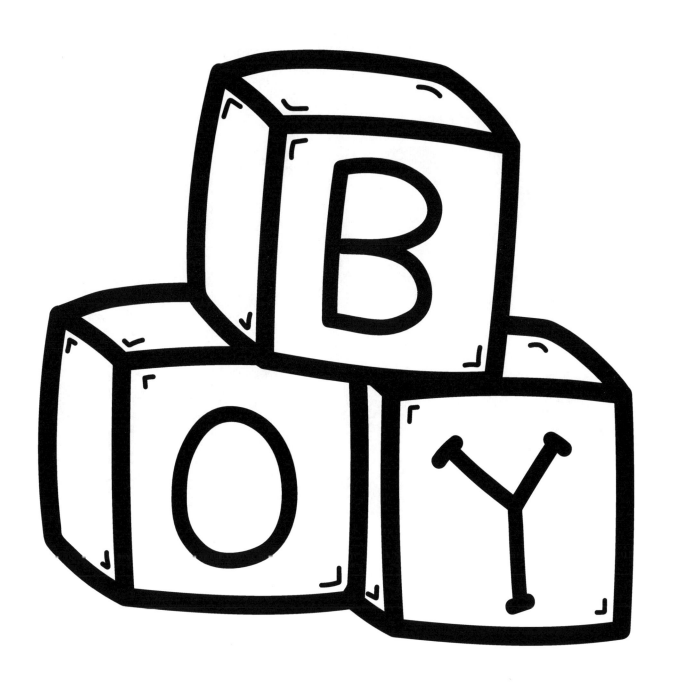

Hello BABY

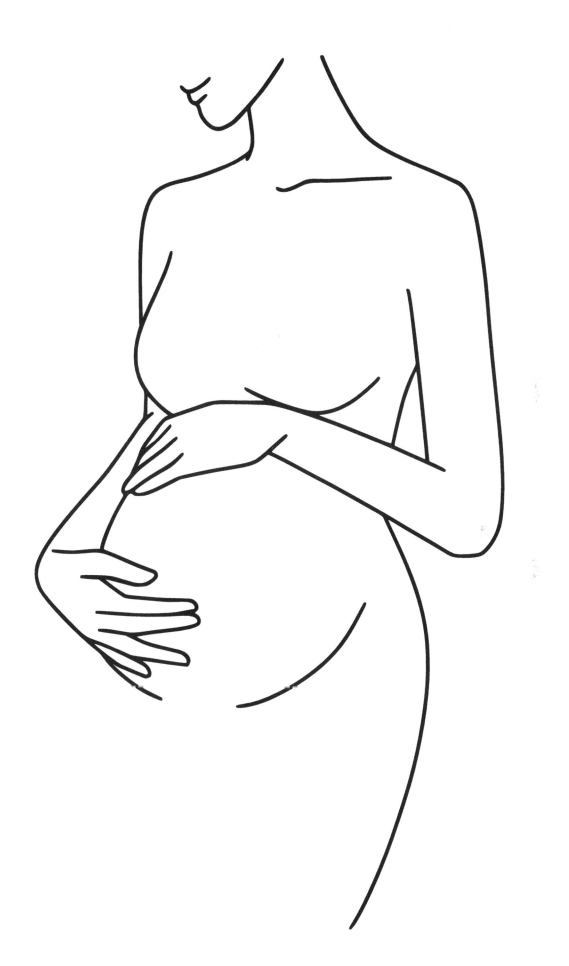

At times your pregnancy can be overwhelming with dr. appointments, weight changes, shift in hormones, cravings, fatigue, illness etc. Where will you enforce healthy boundaries to ensure that you are taking care of yourself mentally and, physically?

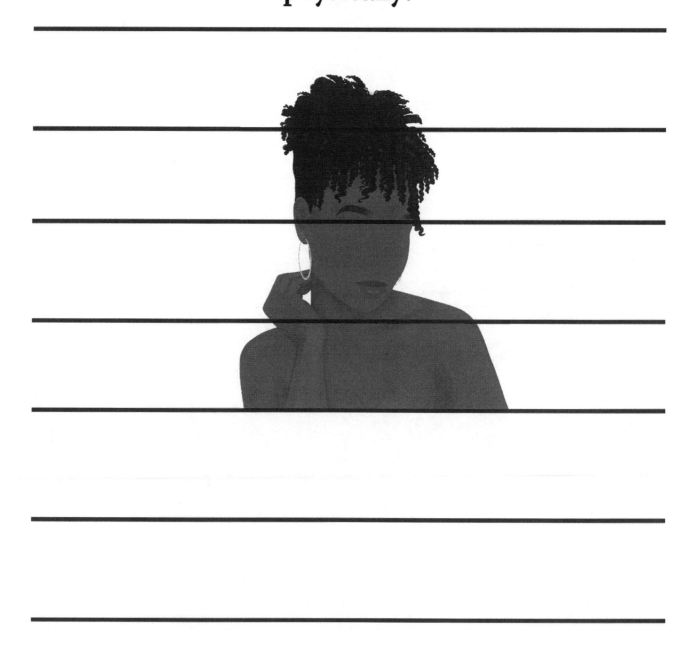

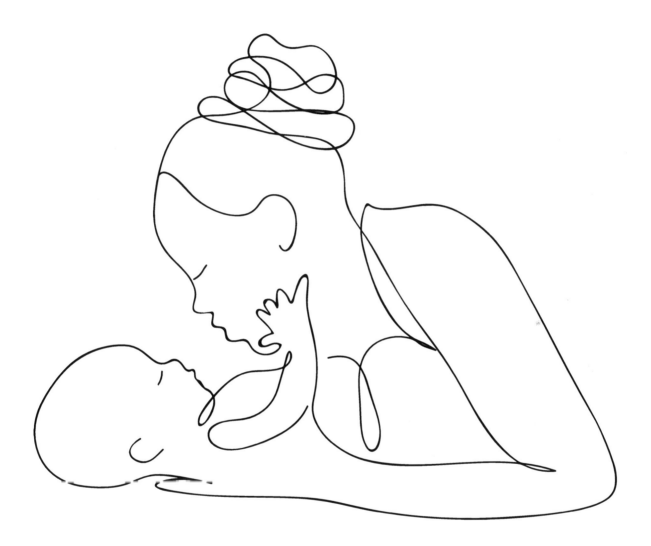

oh baby

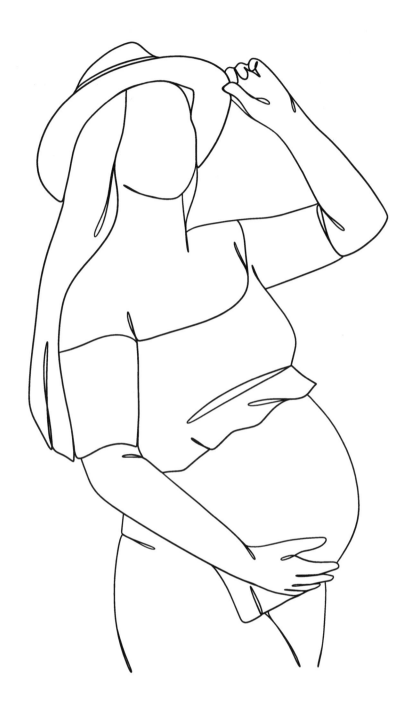

"Embrace the art of stillness, for within it resides the power to nurture life and the beautiful essence of your own being."
Dominique M. Williams

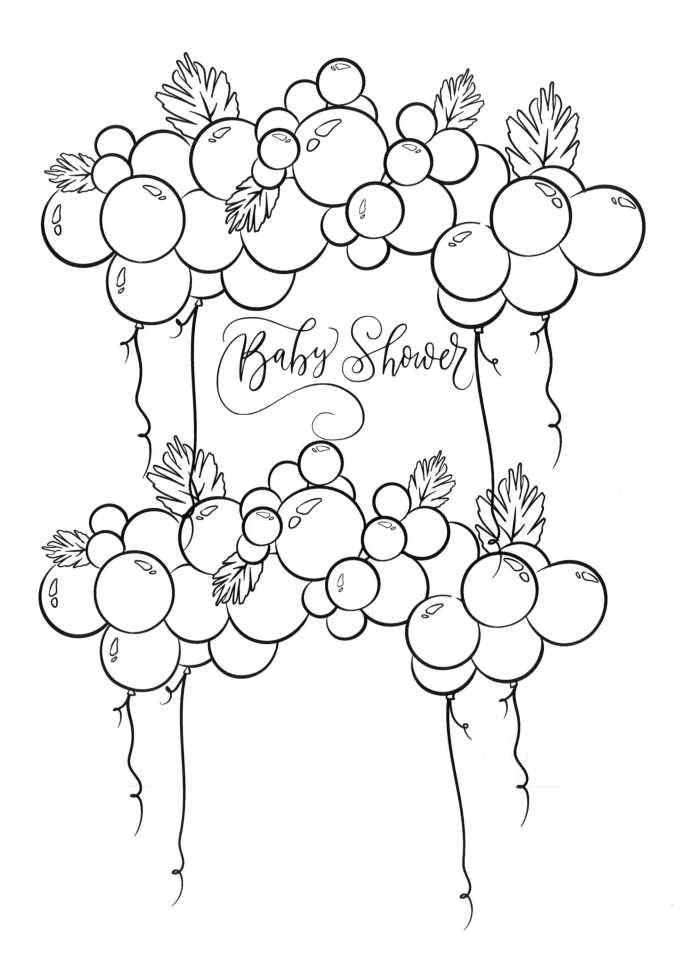

hello little one

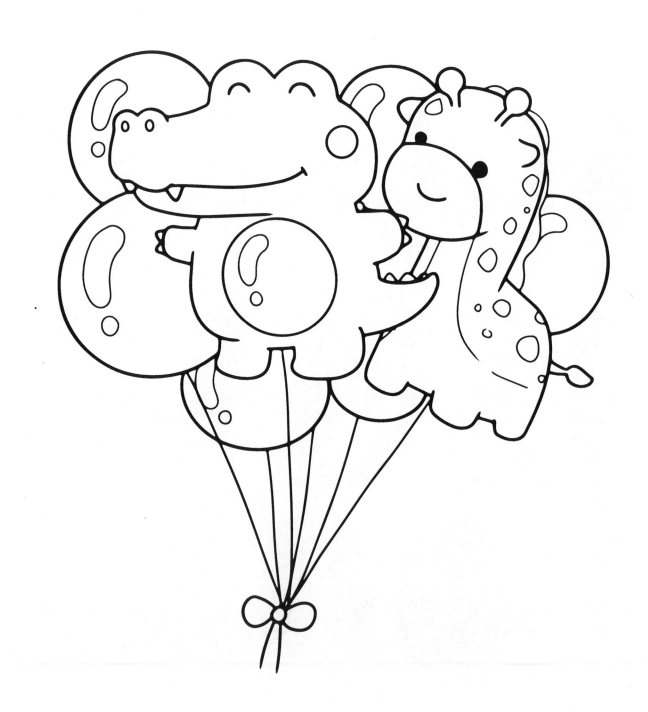

Relax

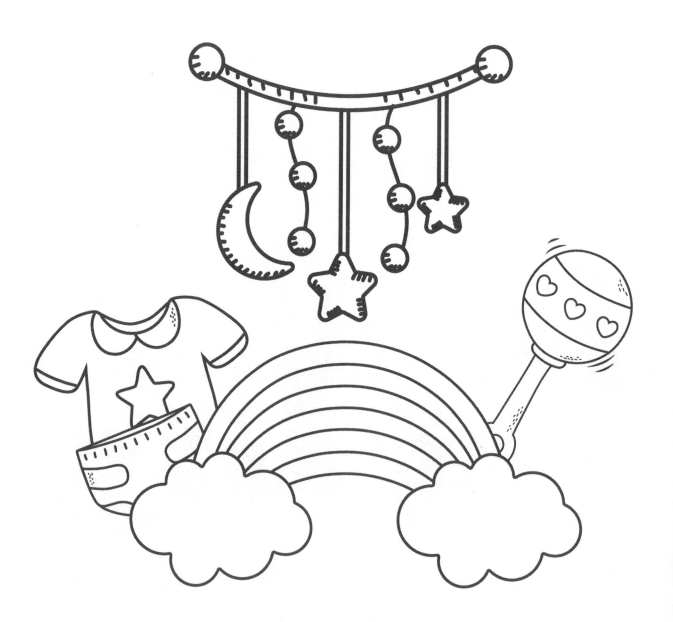

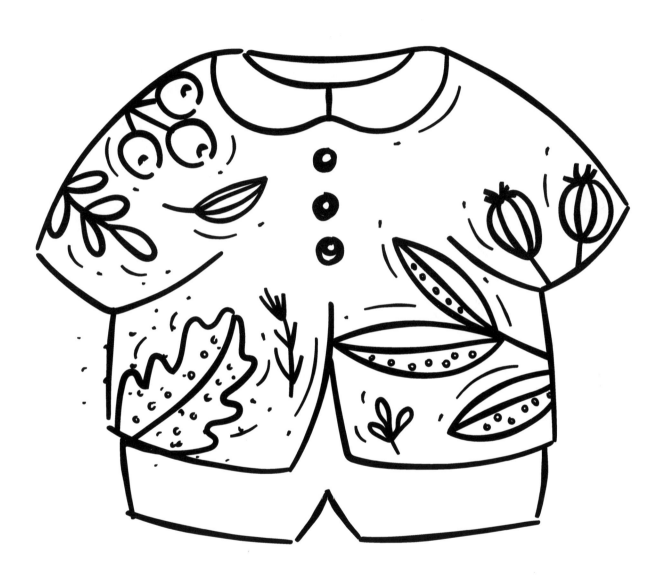

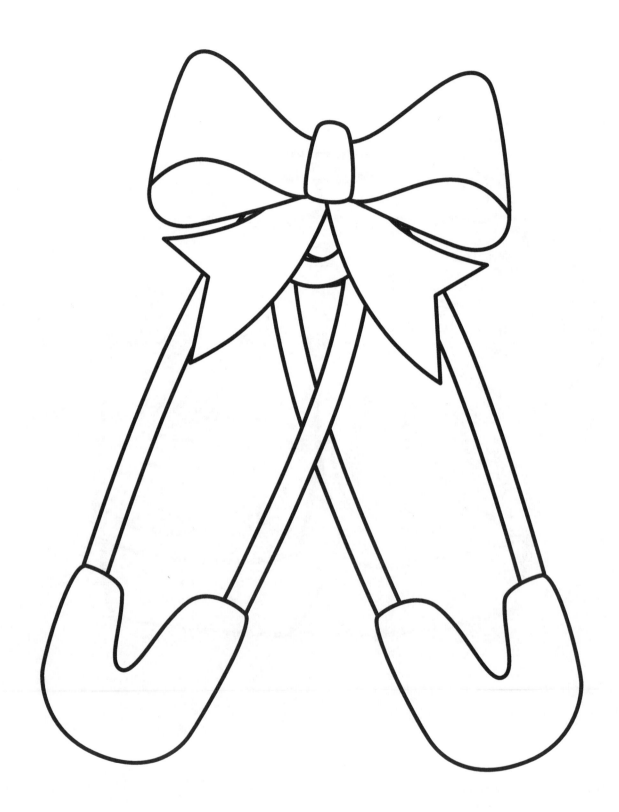

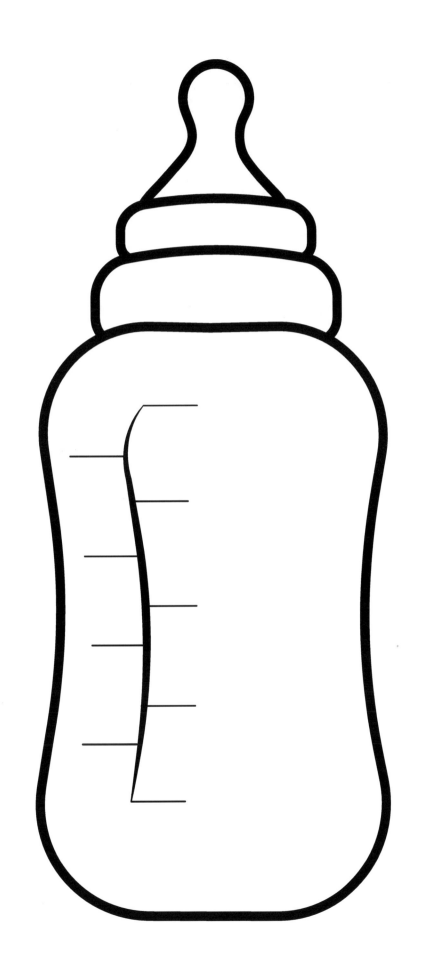

HELLO gorgeous

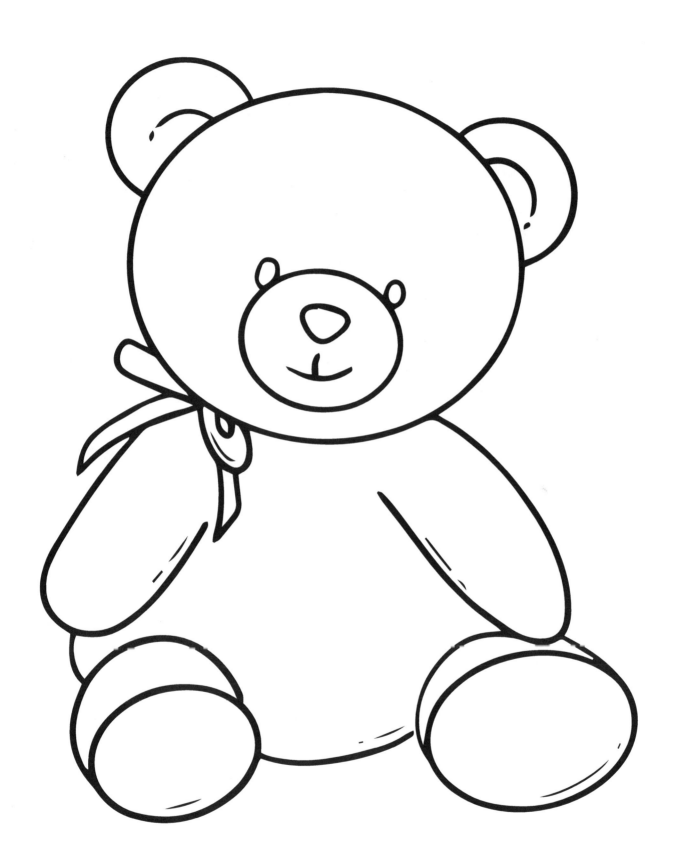

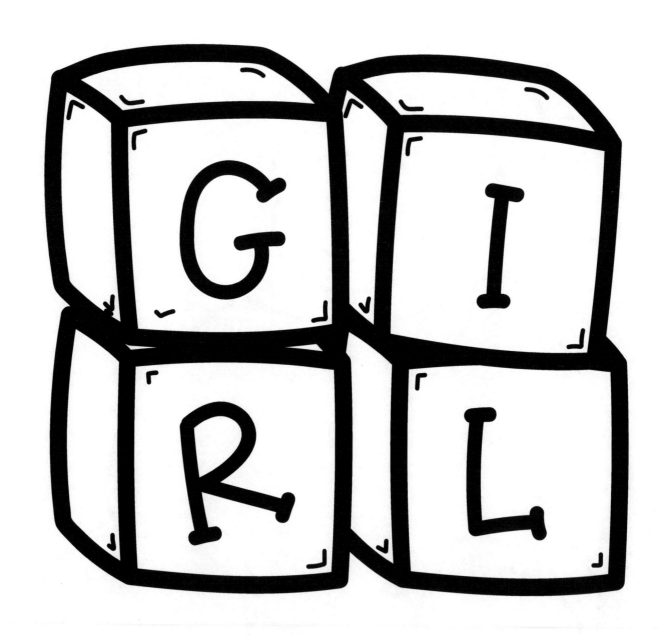

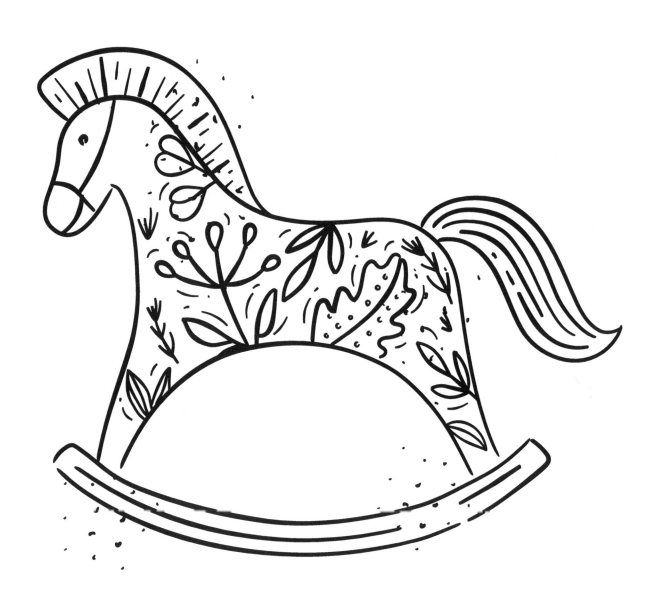

Write your baby a letter.

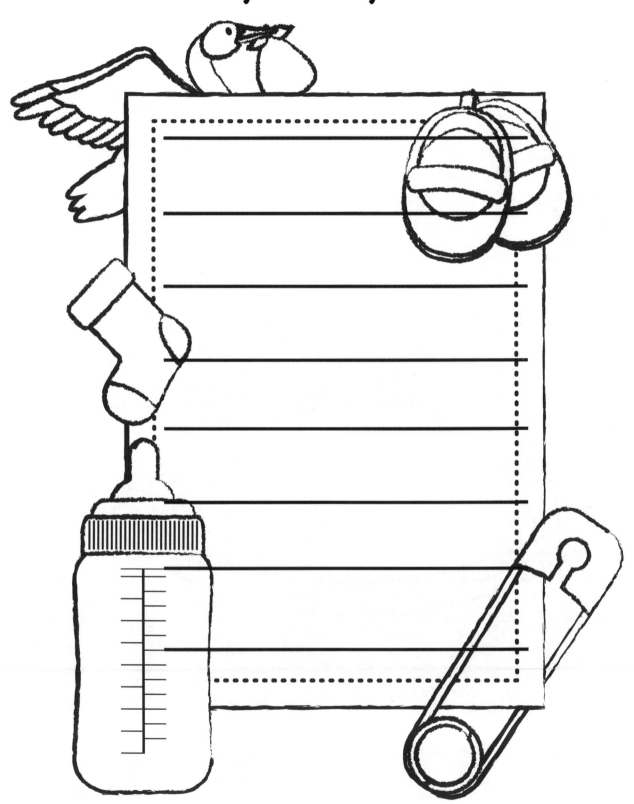

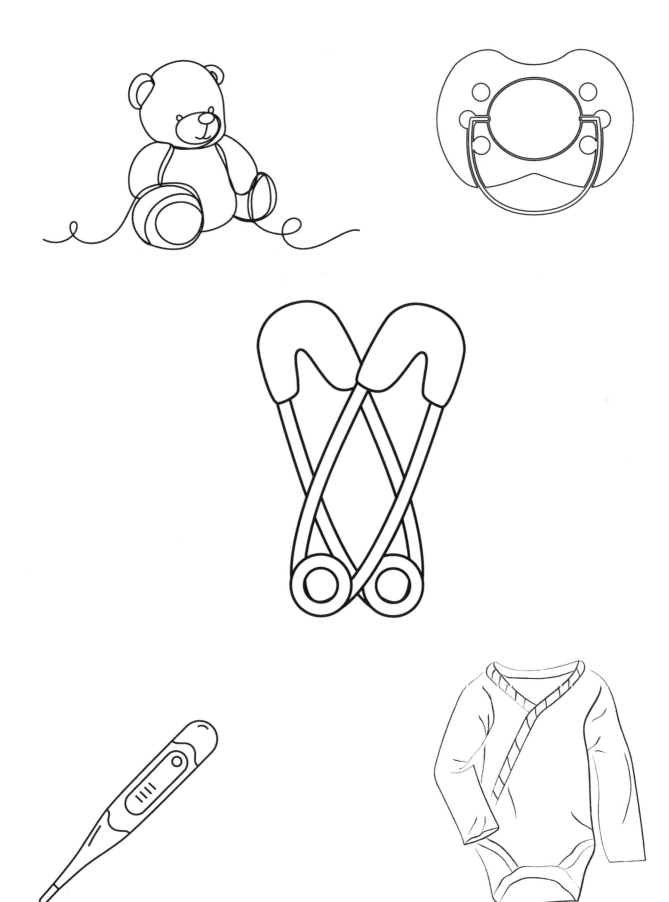

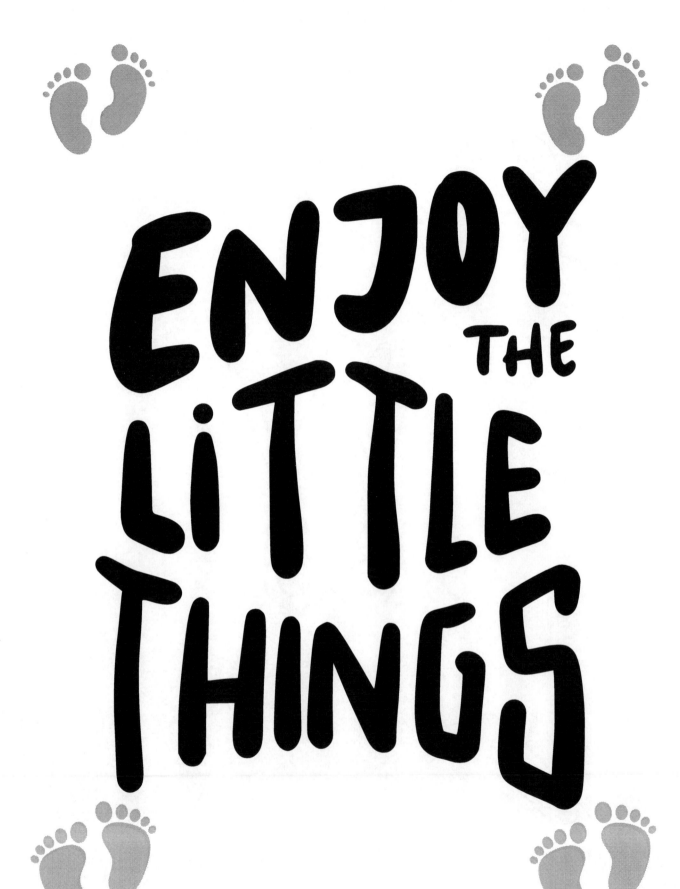

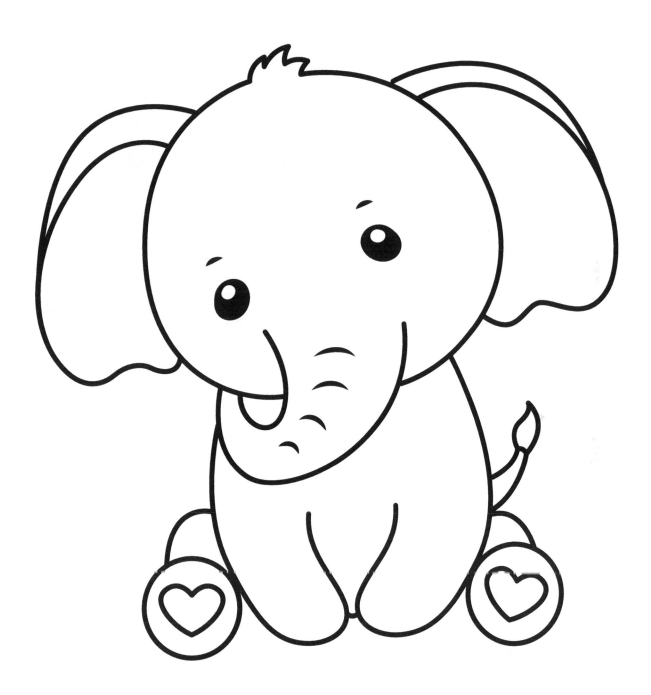

you can do hard things

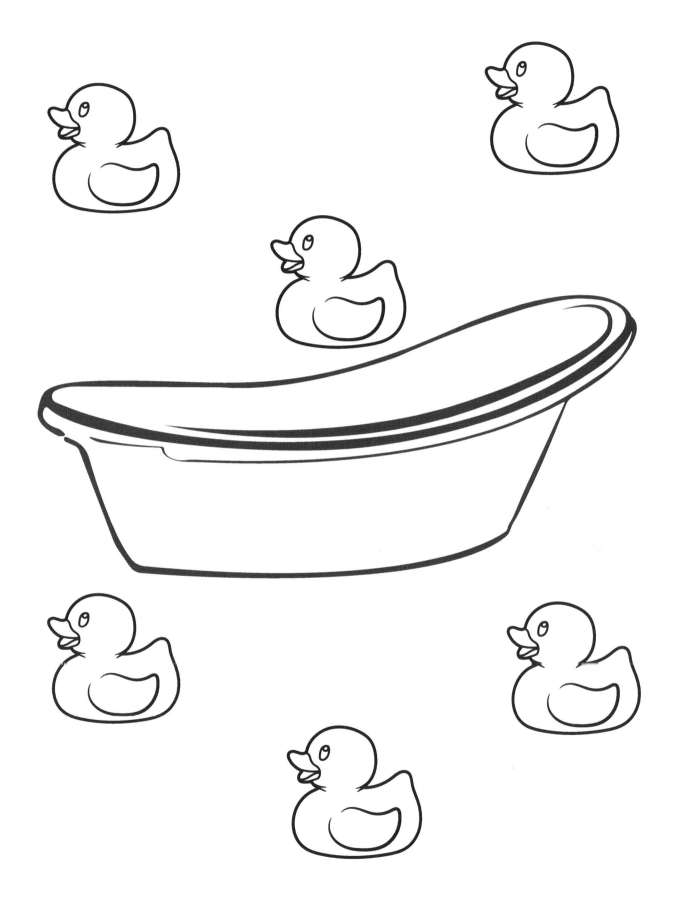

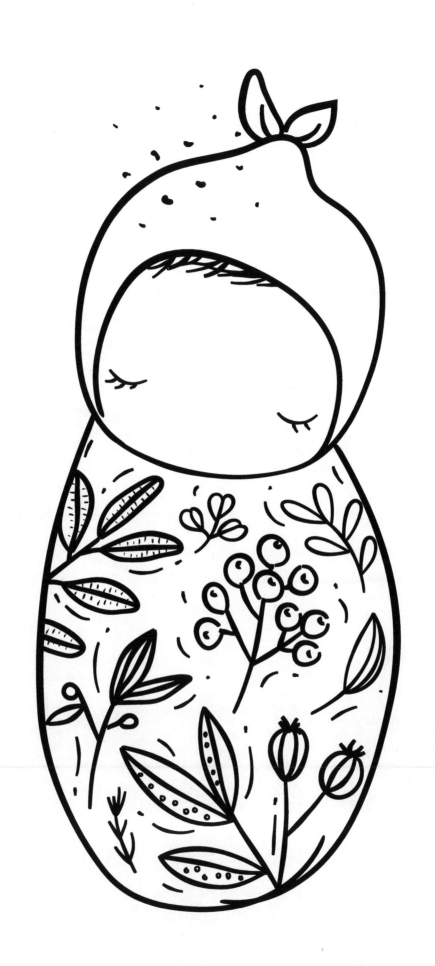

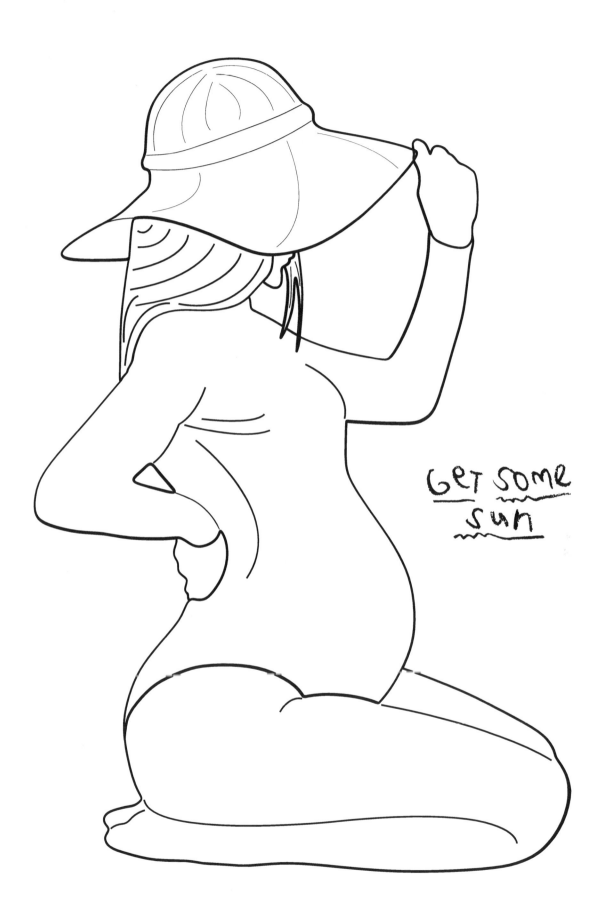

GET SOME
SUN

time to hydrate

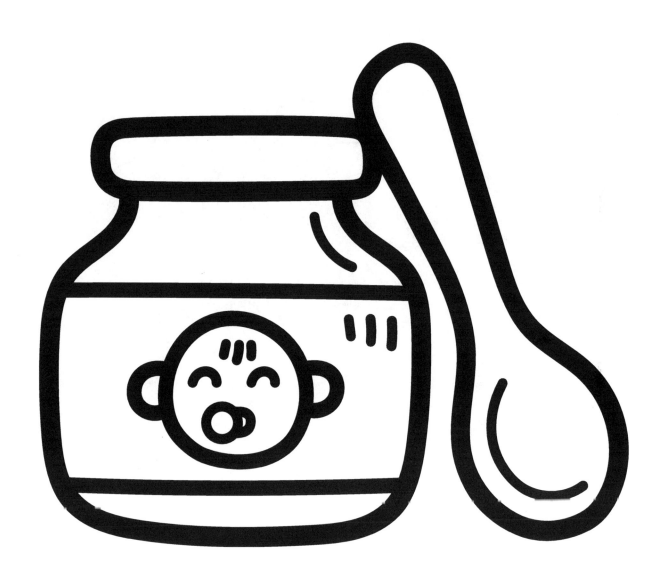

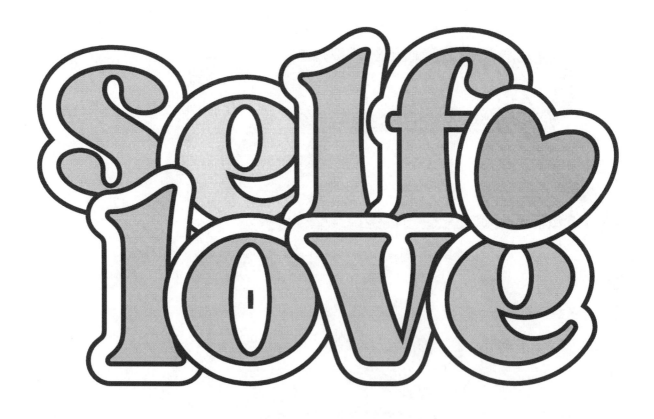

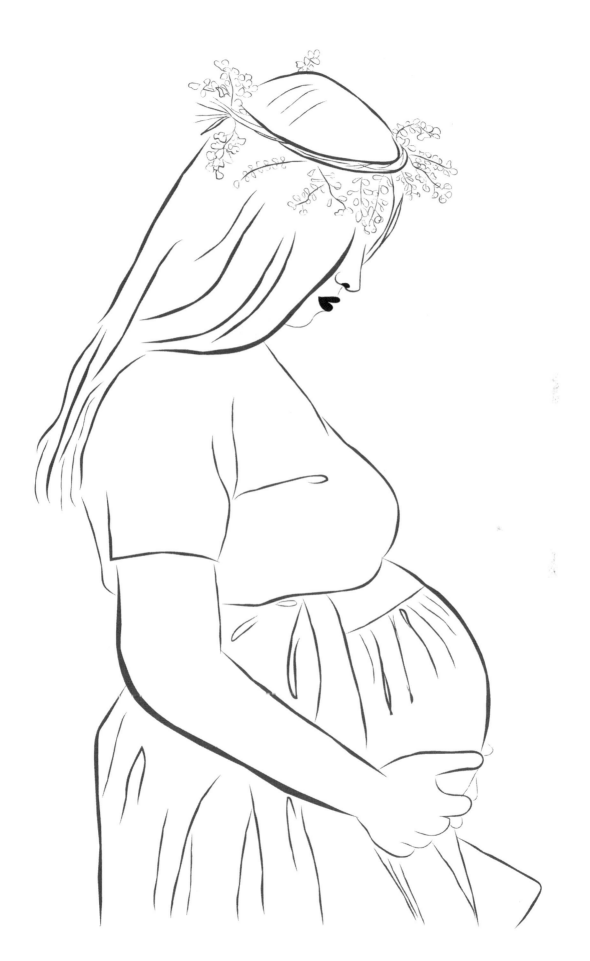

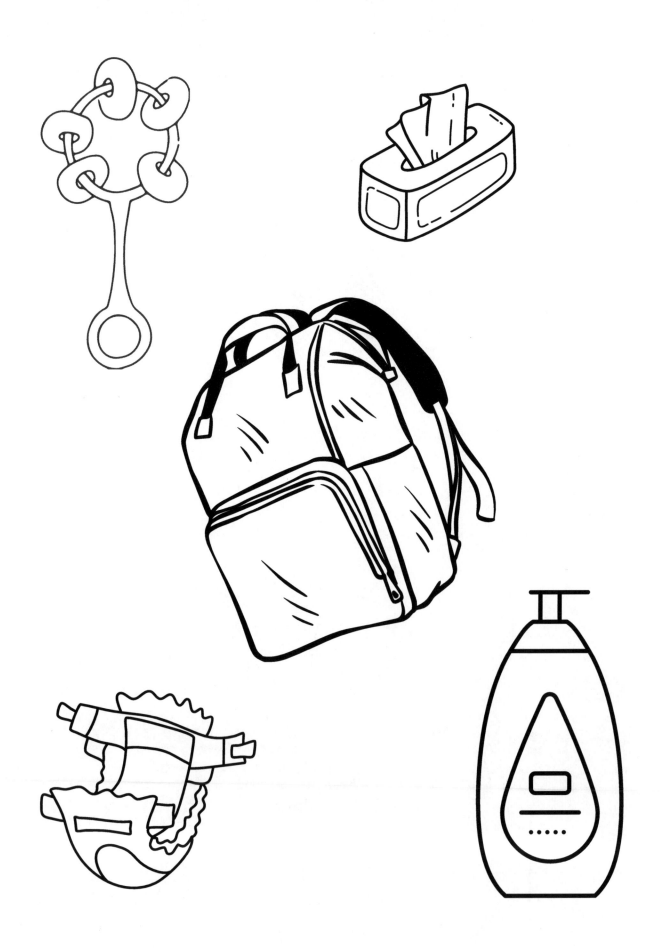

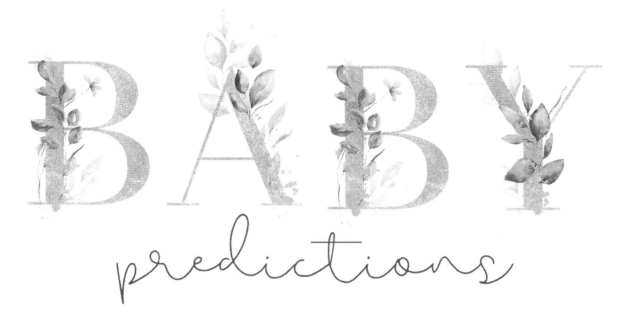

BABY
predictions

Gender

Baby's Name

Date of Birth

Eye Color

Weight

Hair Color

Height

Time of Birth

Parent Qualities:

Love

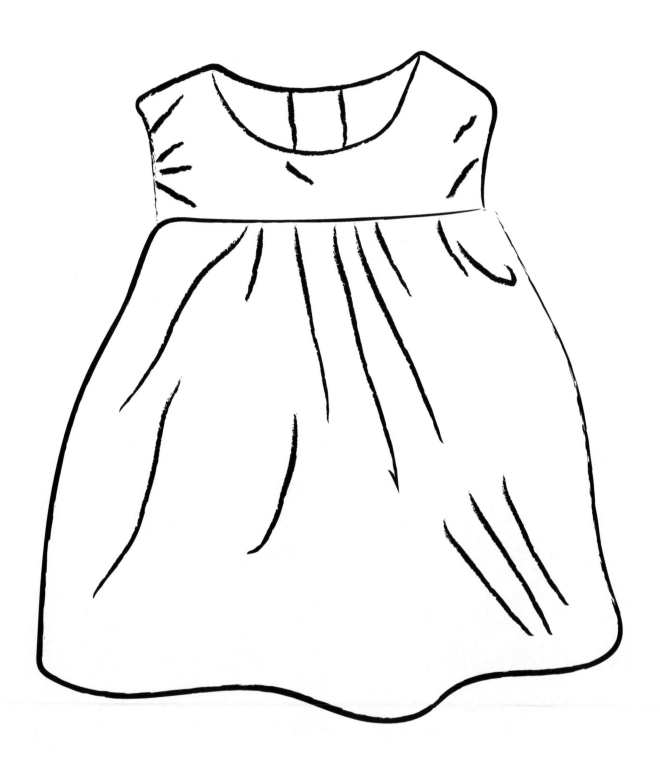

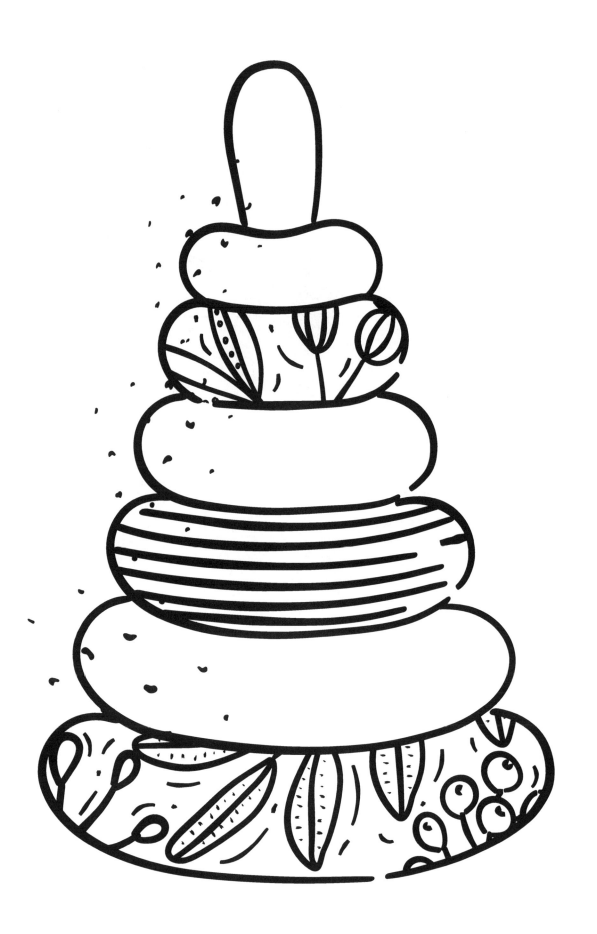

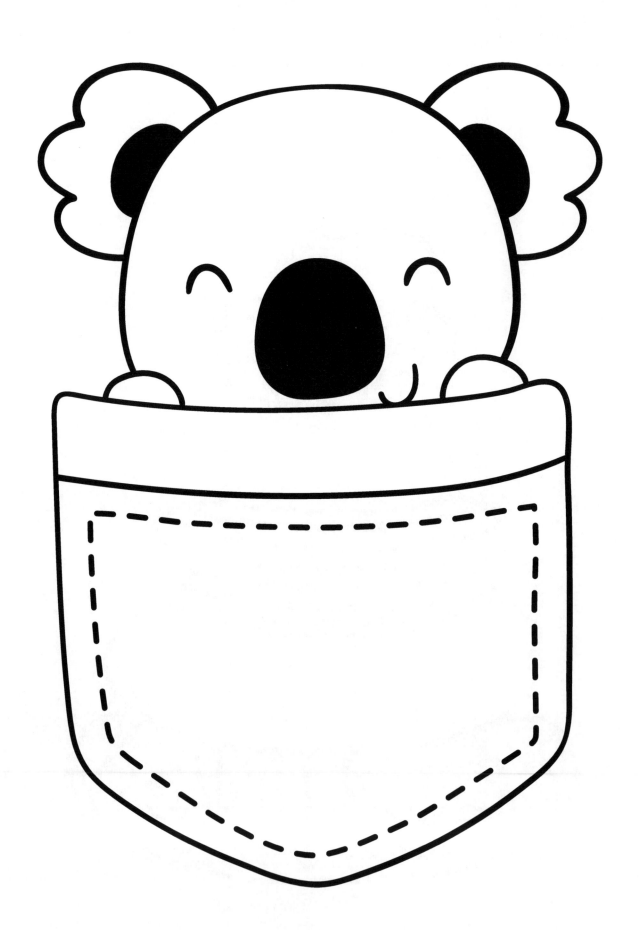

BUT FIRST
Skin care

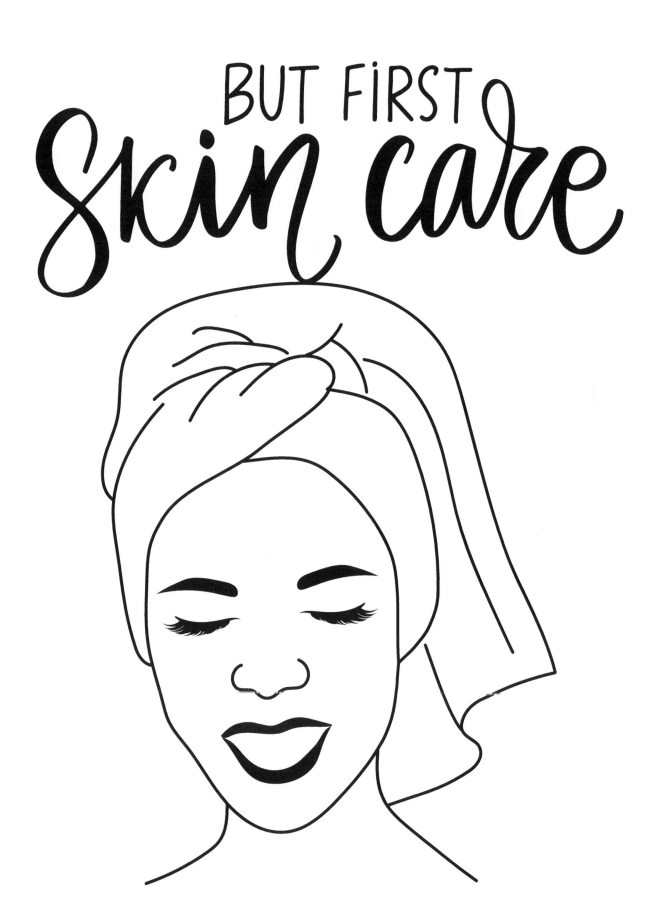

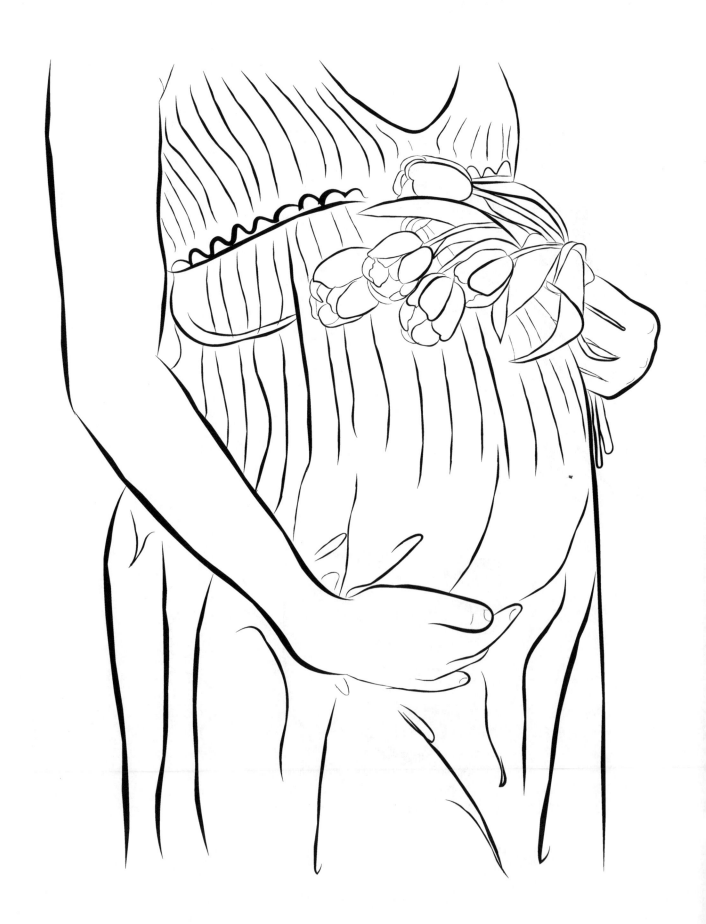

Stronger THAN Yesterday

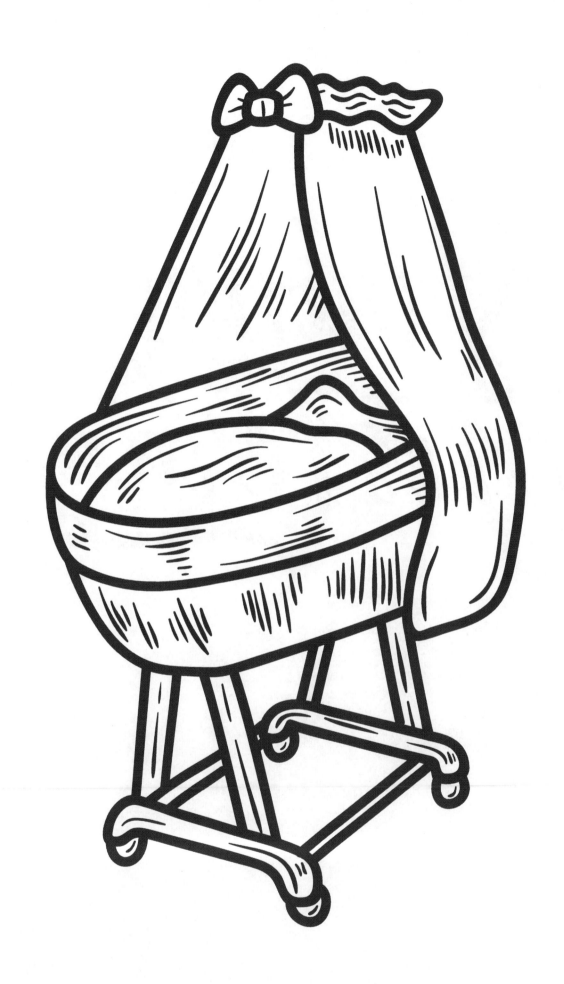

You are strong

BABY GIRL NAMES

a _____

b _____

c _____

d _____

e _____

f _____

g _____

h _____

i _____

j _____

k _____

l _____

m

n _____

o _____

p _____

q _____

r _____

s _____

t _____

u _____

v _____

w _____

x _____

y _____

z

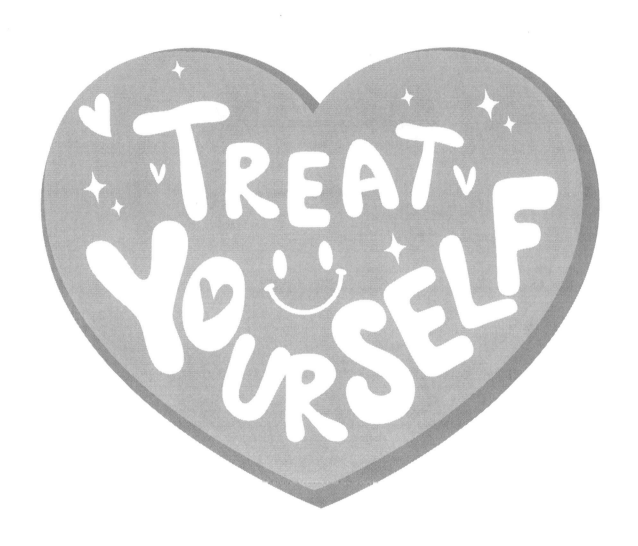

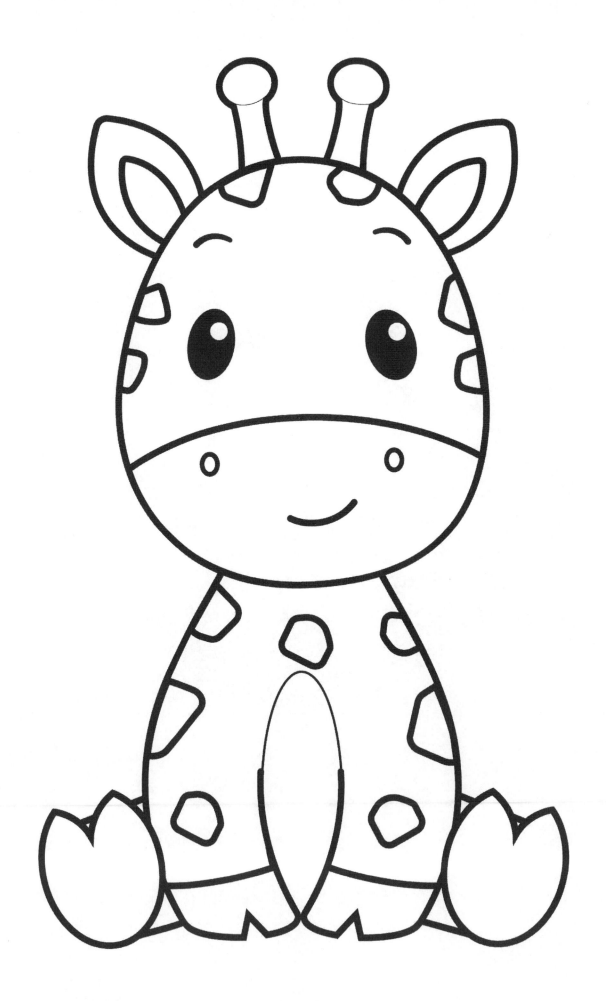

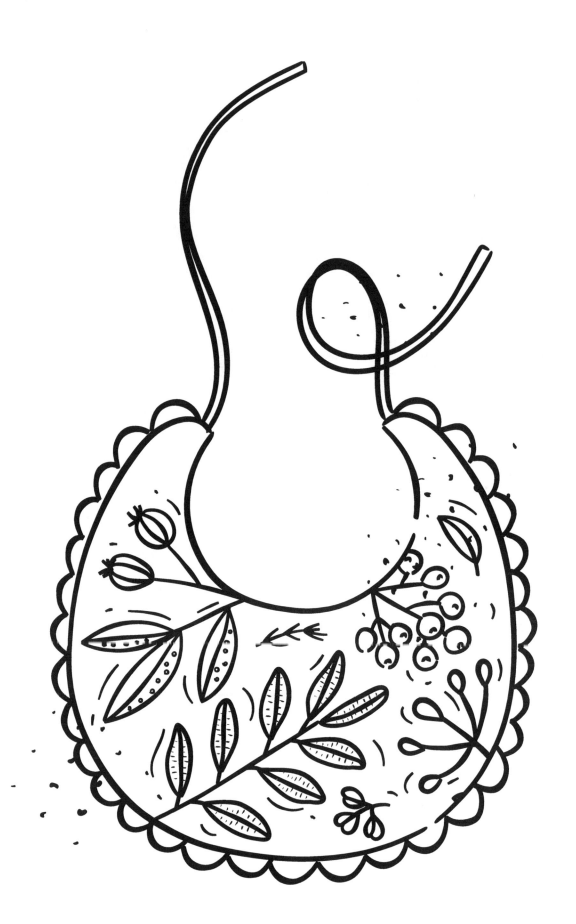

GOOD THINGS TAKE TIME

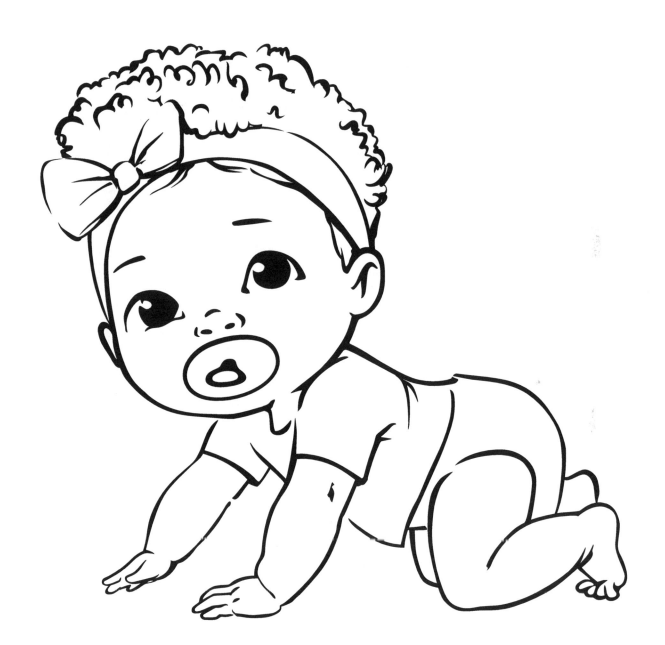

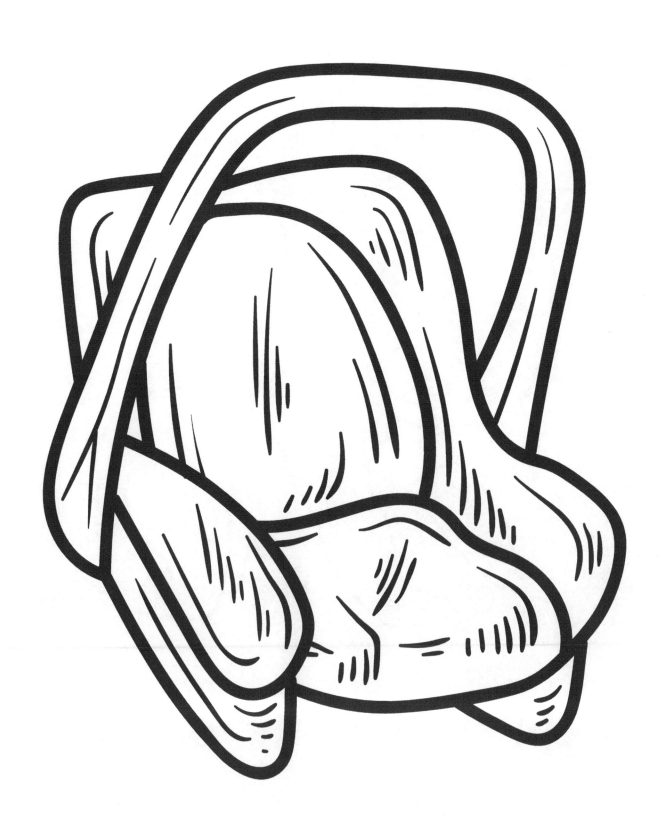

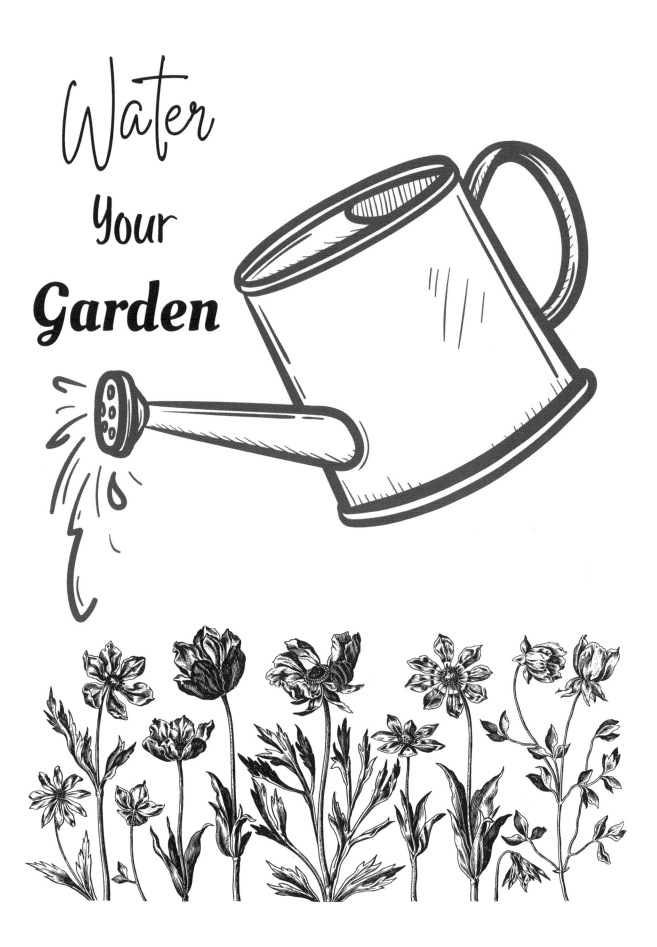

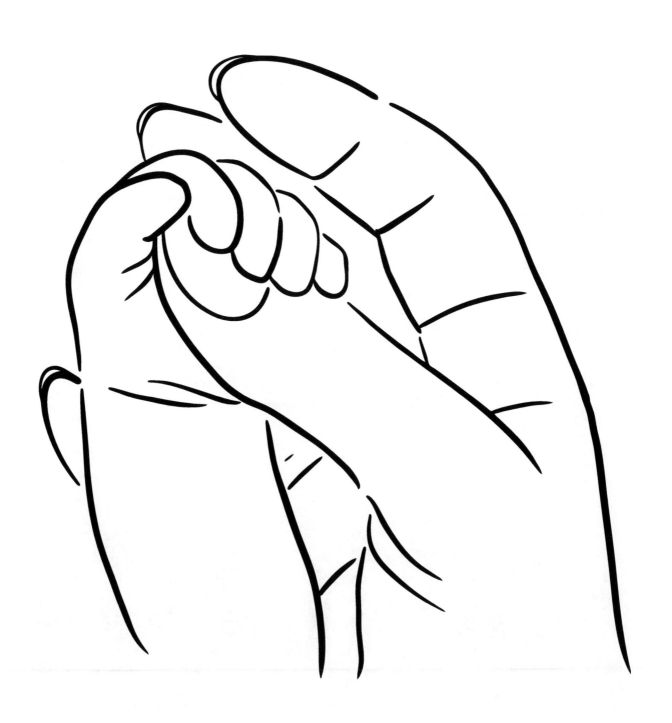

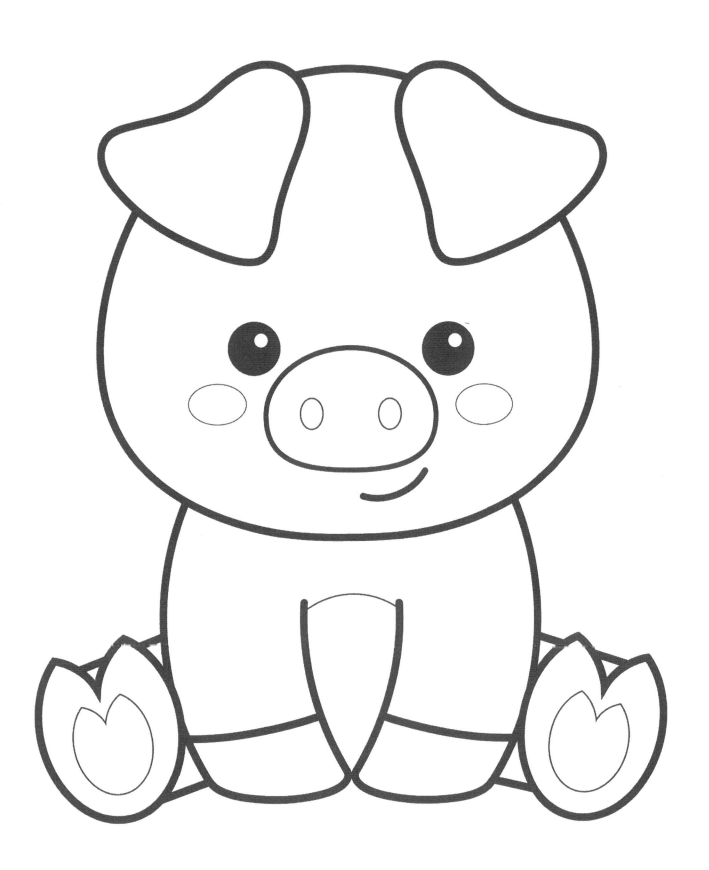

I deserve good things

"Amongst the kicks and flutters, be sure to find moments to pamper your soul."
Dominique M. Williams

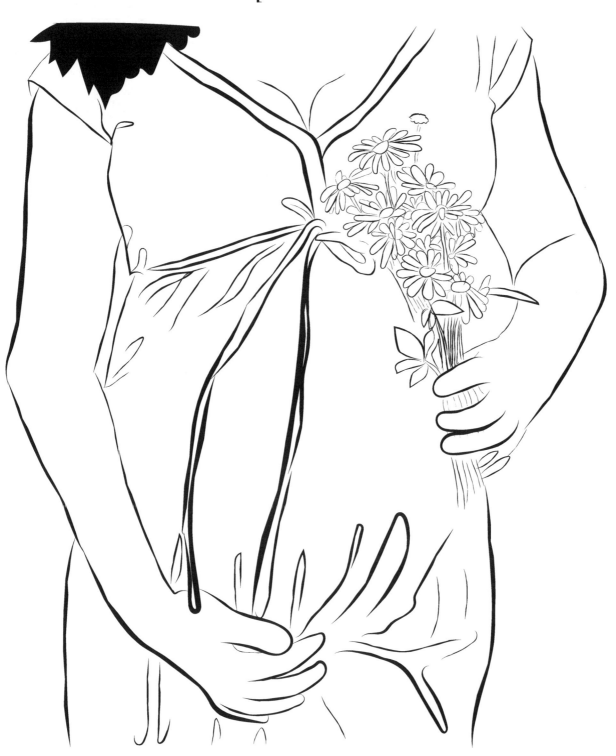

BABY

wishes

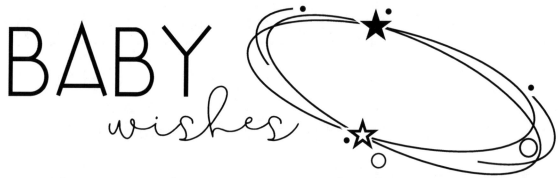

I hope you have your mother's

I hope you have your father's

I hope you grow up to be

I hope you have the character strength of

I hope you become

I hope you are

Love

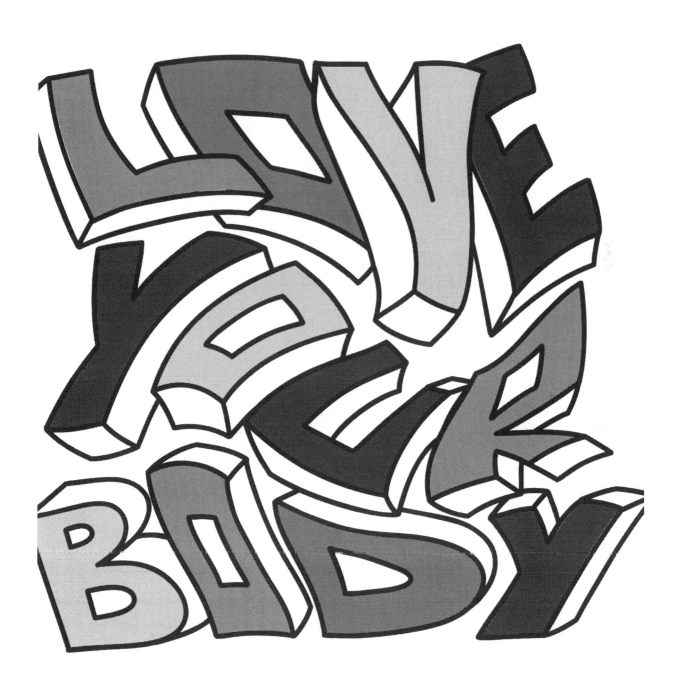

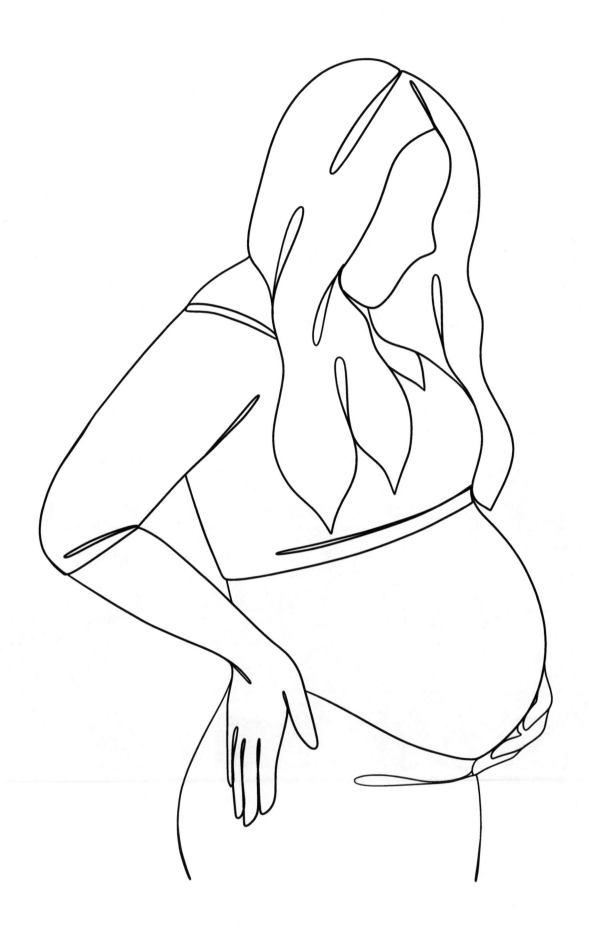

breathe

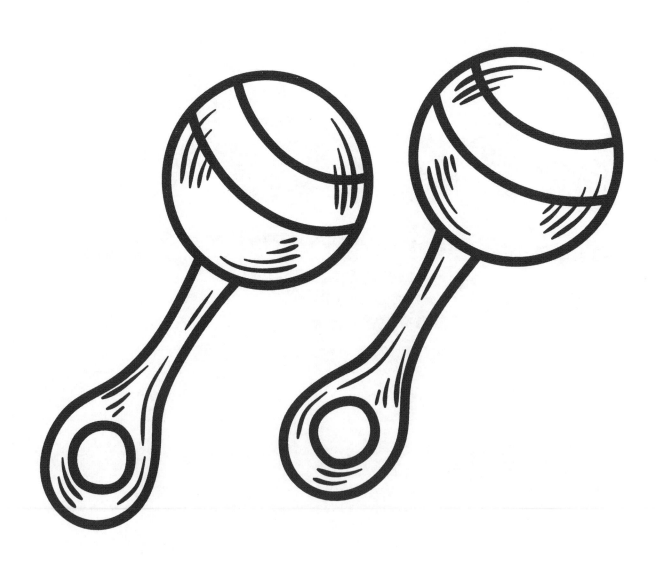

BABY BOY NAMES

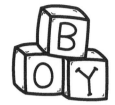

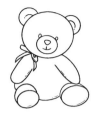

a _____

b _____

c _____

d _____

e _____

f _____

g _____

h _____

i _____

j _____

k _____

l _____

m

n _____

o _____

p _____

q _____

r _____

s _____

t _____

u _____

v _____

w _____

x _____

y _____

z

Breastfeeding may present some challenges consider taking classes during pregnancy and remember to give yourself grace.

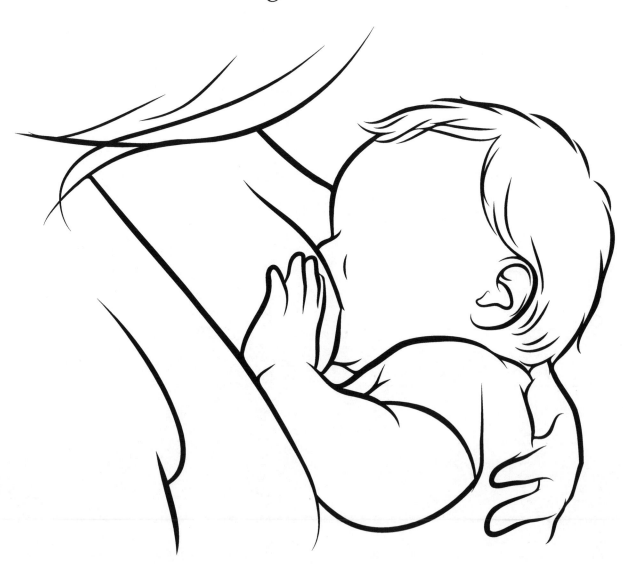

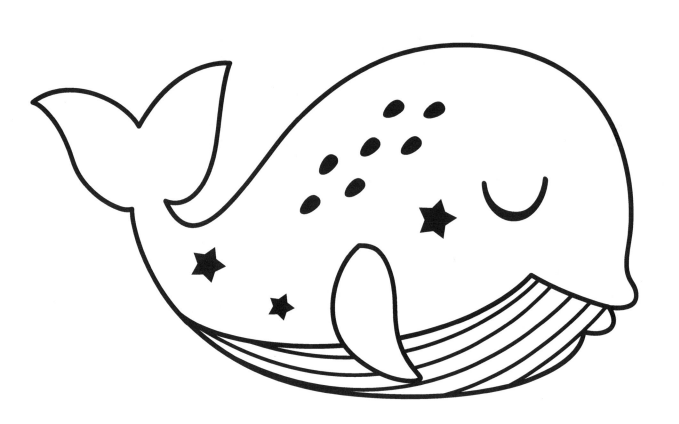

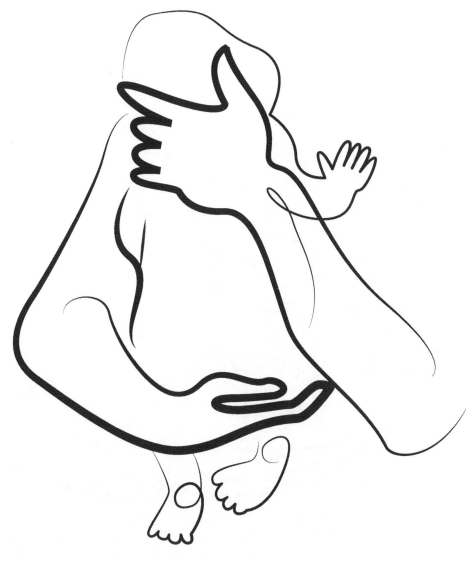

happy mothers day

I am beautiful

A - Z
all things baby!

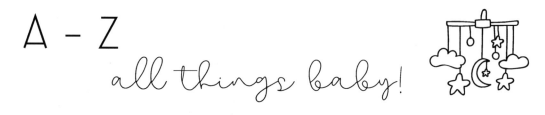

Think of a baby-related item that begins with each letter of the alphabet.

a

b

c

d

e

f

g

h

i

j

k

l

m

n

o

p

q

r

s

t

u

v

w

x

y

z

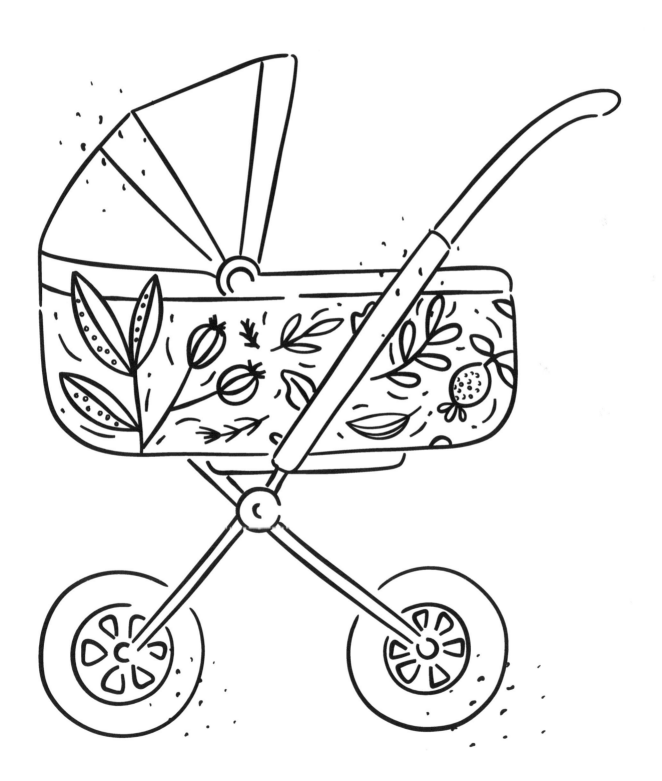

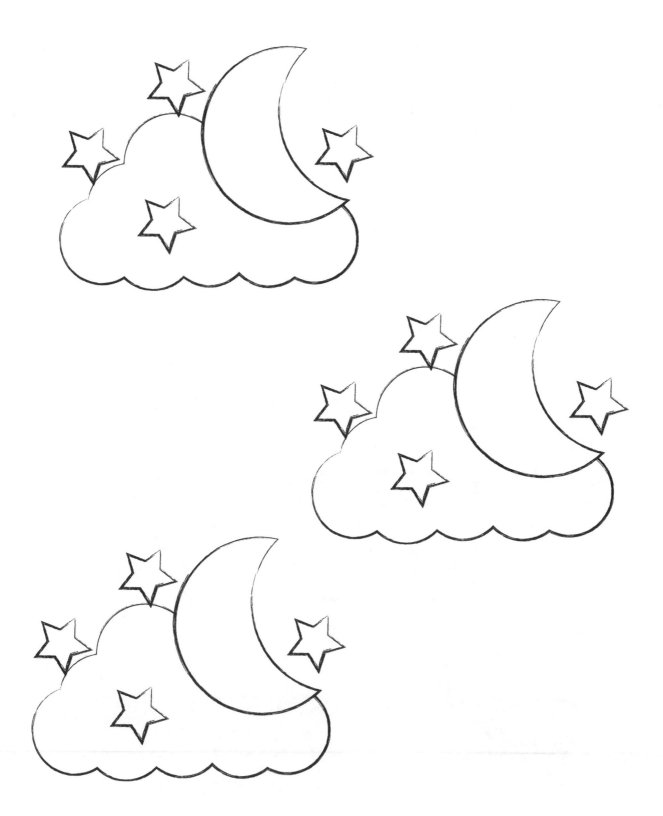

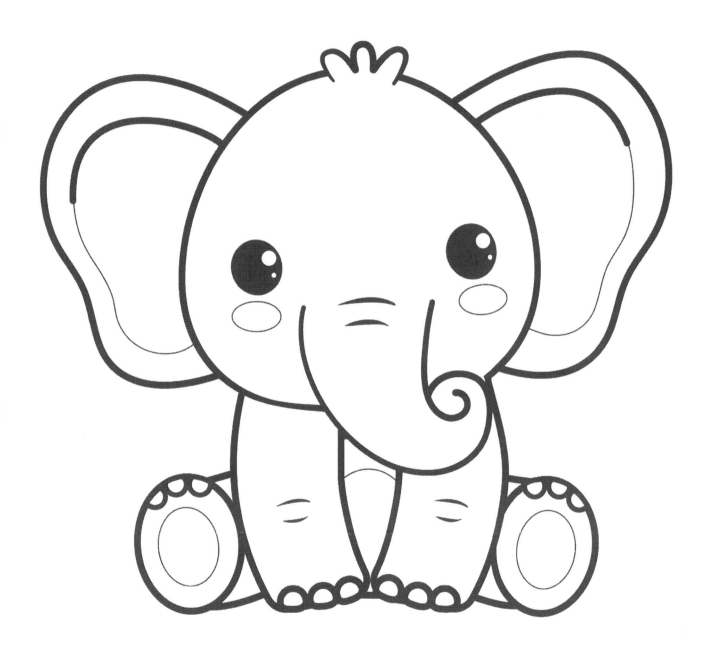

YOU CAN!*

TEAM
BOY

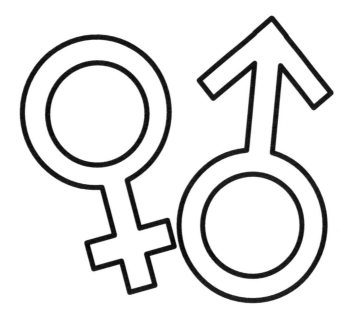

TEAM
GIRL

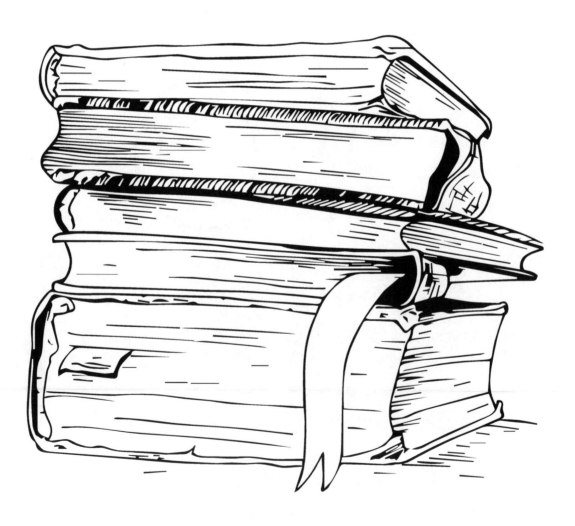

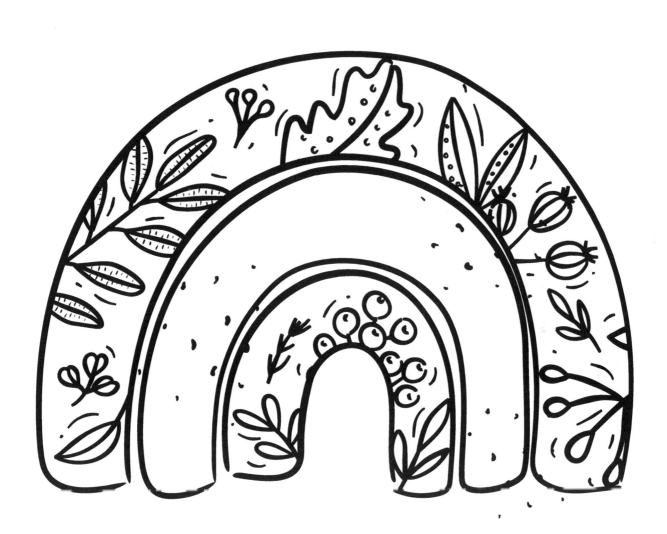

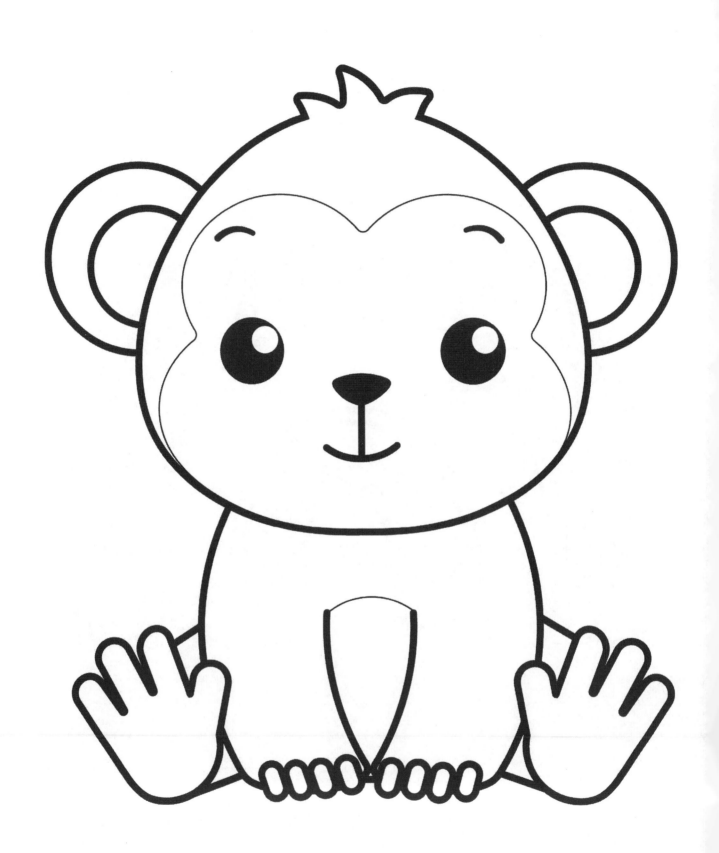

MORE SELFLOVE

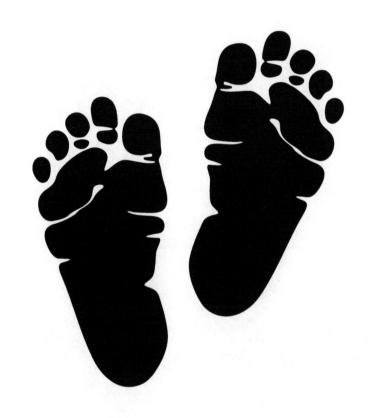

Made in the USA
Columbia, SC
20 April 2024